The Sirtfo

A Diet Plan that gives chocolate and red wine to burn fat, lose weight and Get lean

By

Jessica Davidson

Table of Content

Introduction

Fresh Year, Fresh You, this is typically a scale-induced hysteria accompanied by a diet of hunger. But how about a 'diet' offering weight reduction, muscle recovery, and well-being by balanced nutrition and daily treatments?

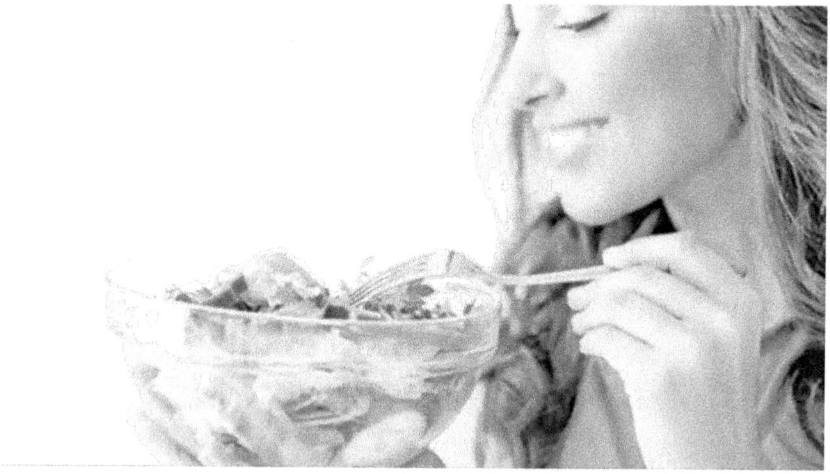

Year after year brings a whole new slimming diet, and this year many of the eye-grabbing stories have been about one that allows you to eat healthily and tastefully - even indulge in chocolate and red wine - without counting calories, while losing weight and staying away from many age ravages.

Sounds too lovely to be real, we agree, but the Sirtfood Diet already has millions of fans with red wine and dark chocolate on the menu and is poised to take the world of diet by storm.

Body acceptance is among the few best things on the internet that have trended for quite some time now. Loving and appreciating ourselves is the motto that most of us seek to obey and give back to our bodies, everything that profoundly loves and preserves us. While enjoying your body is vital; taking care of it and staying safe is equally important. And thanks to the increasing awareness about metabolism and health, diets come up every day that can help us not just keep in shape but also be mentally and emotionally healthy. Once again, one such diet has arisen called the diet of Sirtfood.

Although some dietary habits try to restrict food types or nutrients, some are focusing on the body's holistic well-being. Specific fad diets in the fitness and wellness network perform loops.

In recent years, the Sirtfood diet has been as conventional as the Cabbage Soup Diet, the 5.2 diets, and the Dukan diet, not only popular with Adele but also with celebrities such as Lorraine Pascale and Jodie Kidd. But is it just another diet that offers so much, or does it help you slim down and feel healthier adopting a sirtfood eating plan?

Consumption craze this year is the Sirt diet that helps you to get your cake (well, red wine, and chocolate) and even consume it promising to trigger your skinny genes. Some people take a nutritional road-test that helped British star Adele slim down to see whether they too could search their lean genes for those tight jeans. Wait, so what? Will they have flaky genes? We all do. The UK makers of the diet, fitness experts Aidan Goggins and Glen Matten, say that in seven days you can drop seven pounds (3 kg) if you adhere to their calorie-restricted meal plan with "wonder foods" that trigger the thin genes, or sirtuins (the same fasting-activated fat-burning genes).

Without any need to dedicate to a stiff schedule of exercises on the side.

People who followed this diet explain it as they embark on a sirt diet packed with hope and excitement, their kitchen loaded with red wine, dark chocolate, and green juice ingredients. A week later, they also felt fantastic at the end of "phase one." May it be that foods such as chocolate, cocoa, chili, garlic, walnuts, rocket, and red wine, which trigger sirtuin, worked their magic?

Now, when you head to the grocery store and fill your cart full of Two-Buck Chuck and Hershey's Hugs, a diet like that isn't just as good. The lowdown here is: The Sirtfood diet is based on sirtuins, a family of proteins present in food. Research has shown that food with high amounts of a sirtuin can help muscle growth and fat burn. "Sirtfoods" are necessary foods that activate these specific genes and enable them to function for you. The headline-grabbers for the Sirtfood Diet are red wine and dark chocolate, as these appear to be rich in sirtuin activators.

The goal is not to consume a diet made entirely of such items but to integrate them as much as you can into your meals. For starters, it would be nice to have a smoothie composed of kale, blueberries, strawberries, and a splash of turmeric. This may also be an excellent choice for those of you java lovers out there because this is one diet that promotes the morning cup of juice.

The Sirtfood Diet has two phases that last three weeks altogether. You will then proceed to "sirtify" your diet by adding as many sirt items as possible into your meals.

Interestingly, coffee is another top sirtfood, which is good news if you're fed up being advised to remove caffeine. Countries where citizens still eat a large number of sirt foods like Japan and Italy, both of which are consistently ranked as the healthiest countries in the world.

The program promises that in seven days, the members will drop seven pounds, "because they feel sustainable strength and consume all the foods you enjoy."

Sounds crazy? We think so, too. Mainly when they discuss "foods that we love." Foods such as spinach, dark chocolate, beer, red wine, and champagne.

Such foods (and drinks) are high in polyphenols (antioxidants) and activate the sirtuin enzyme according to the Sirtfood Diet, which is believed to have a beneficial impact on the metabolism, mood, and may slow down the signs of aging.

While there is no doubt that an antioxidant-rich diet is right for you, there is still some discussion as to whether or not sirtuins are responsible for the health-promoting benefits of antioxidant-rich food.

With many celebrities publicly supporting and professing the benefits of other foods, a sirtfood diet is the one diet that has drawn the interest of others.

There is also an increasing range of celebrity fans of the Sirtfood Diet, including Adele, Jodie Kidd, Lorraine Pascale, and Sir Ben Ainslie.

Sports personalities such as Olympic gold medalist Ben Ainslie, British boxer David Haye, and English rugby player James Haskell, who all rely on their bodies performing at their best, have recommended The SirtFood Diet, and not championed by celebrities as a fad diet instead. And, most notably, it is believed that the Sirtfood Diet is the eating program behind the dramatic weight loss of Adele.

Even if this weren't enough to persuade you to check it out, on average, people would lose weight quickly - in reality, seven pounds (3.2 kg) on the Sirtfood Diet in only seven days. Yeah, you read that right; in only one week, this is half a pound!

Correct speaking, many people figured that was made up when they first heard about the diet. And to create more confusion is that spell check insists it isn't even a word. As other stuff in our mad diet business, though, it isn't formulated, and so-called experts consider it the golden cure to weight loss.

So, to clear all those doubts about the sirtfood diet and have a detailed knowledge of this latest diet trend, continue reading the book. All the questions in your head about this diet would be clearly answered and explained in this book, and by the time you finish reading this book, you would be able to decide whether this diet is for you or not. We'll find out in this book if this lifestyle is the be-all and end-all diets and what proof remains to back up this.

So buckle up, and start your journey of sirtfood diet.

Chapter 1: Introduction to Sirtood Diet

Instead of promoting starvation and shame over calorie consumption, The Sirtfood Diet is overusing 'wonder foods' to turbocharge your body not just to maximize weight loss, but also to boost your overall long-term health.

The Sirtfood diet focuses on sirtuin-rich diets, or SIRT1-SIRT7.

Sirtuins are known to help control fat and glucose metabolism in response to energy level changes. These proteins also impact calorie restriction on aging changes. The diet is said to affect the body's ability to burn fat and boost the metabolic system.

Before starting the diet, you should know some basics of the sirtfood diet discussed in the upcoming units of this chapter.

1.1 Defining Sirtfood Diet

Sirtfoods are (pretty recently revealed) diets plan with types of food that activate the 'sirtuin' genes in our body, and the genes activated in fasting diets. The book lists top sirtfoods including birds-eye chill, buckwheat, capers, celery, chocolate, green tea, and kale and details a 21-day diet plan that is very high in the top 20 Sirtfoods.

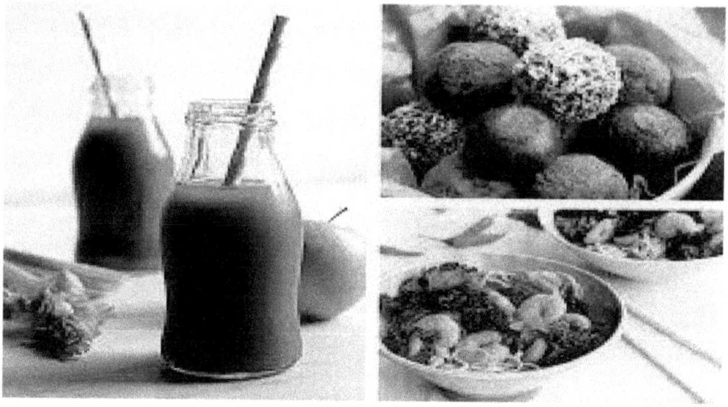

The science behind the diet is focused on these Sirtfoods, a group of newly discovered regular plant foods rich in a chemical compound known as 'sirtuin' activators.

These sirtuin activators are a protein type that activates the body's so-called 'skinny gene' pathways.

These narrow pathways are more generally triggered by fasting and exercise and help the body lose fat, increase muscle mass, and improve health. Countries where people eat a significant number of Sirtfoods as part of their conventional diet, like Japan and Italy, are consistently ranked among the world's healthiest countries.

What sounds like a snack taken straight from a sci-fi movie, is a food rich in sirtuin activators, says nutritionist Rob Hobson. Sirtuins are a type of protein that prevents our cells from dying or being inflamed by disease, but research has shown that they can help control your metabolism, increase muscle, and burn fat - hence the new 'wonder food' name.

According to diet creators, these particular foods function by activating different proteins in the body called sirtuins. Sirtuins are believed to prevent body cells from dying while under stress and are thought to control inflammation, metabolism, and aging. Sirtuins are believed to affect the body's ability to burn fat and improve metabolism, resulting in a seven-pound weight loss a week while retaining muscle. However, some researchers say this is unlikely to be a purely fat loss but may also reflect improvements in skeletal muscle and liver glycogen stocks.

The research behind Sirtfoods comes from a 2003 study that found a compound present in red wine increased yeast lifespan. Ultimately, this led to research illustrating the health benefits of red wine, and how (if moderately drunk) people who consume red wine acquire little weight.

Almost all of the theory behind the Sirtfood diet plan is close to that 'fasting diets' that have been common for the past couple of years, whereby our bodies trigger genes, and our fat storage is turned off; our bodies mostly switch to survival mode, hence weight loss. Weak to fasting-diets are the unavoidable hunger that results in energy depletion, irritable actions (when you're "hungry"), exhaustion, and muscle weakness. The Sirtfood diet claims to combat these negatives because it's not easy, so hunger isn't an issue, making it ideal for those who would like to live a healthier lifestyle.

To us carnivores, the protein is essential to maintain metabolism and minimize muscle loss in the diet. Leucine, an amino acid found in protein, reinforces, and strengthens Sirtfoods' behavior. The best way to eat Sirtfoods is to pair them with a chicken breast, steak, or other leucine sources such as fish or eggs.

Sirtfood diet is based on SIRT or sirtuin science. According to a study by Glenn Laboratory for Aging Science, Massachusetts, they are a category of seven proteins present in the human body, including metabolism, inflammation, and lifespan.

The sirtfood diet works on the assumption that some plant compounds may increase these proteins. These are dubbed sirtfoods.

Combining sirt foods with calorie restriction may cause the body to produce higher sirtuin levels, leading to rapid weight loss while maintaining muscle mass.

Sirtuins are a protein class found in living organisms involving metabolic processes. 'Sirtfoods' are rich in sirtuin modulators, imitating diet and workout results by burning fat, increasing muscle, and staining off disease. According to Aidan Goggins and Glen Matten, the pioneers of the Sirtfood Diet, storing sirtuin-rich foods like kale, green tea, and apples, will activate the 'skinny' gene pathways and help you lose fat quickly.

Sirtfood diet is two-phase-based;

Phase one is an intensive seven-day program to kick-start the severe weight loss.

Then, phase two is about raising the quantity of Sirtfood-rich products in your daily meals to maintain weight loss.

The Sirtfood program, unlike many other short-term yo-yo diets, provides meals and guidance on how to hold off the weight you lose in the first week by incorporating Sirtfoods as part of a safe, balanced diet.

1.2 Origins of Sirtfood Diet

A pair of writers and fitness experts named Aidan Goggins and Glen Matten, who have mostly focused on eating healthy rather than weight loss, introduced the concept of a sirtfood diet. The pair set out a meal plan in their new book, The Sirtfood Diet, which includes drinking three sirtfood green juices a day accompanied by healthy sirtfood-rich meals, such as buckwheat and prawn stir-fry or smoked salmon sirt super salad.

Nutritional scientists Aidan Goggins and Glenn Matten, are doing groundbreaking work into what is now considered sirt foods, which have put out The Sirt Food Diet.

Starting in 2003, researchers found that specific forms of diet include foods that involve substances capable of switching on 'skinny genes' called sirtuins that are usually only triggered while we are fasting and exercising. They are not solely responsible for fat burning and controlling appetite, but also for cell defense and repair, and as such encourage muscle building - most weight loss regimes result in muscle loss - and cardiac health, thus helping to prevent degenerative and inflammatory disorders such as osteoporosis, arthritis, diabetes and probably other cancers.

Goggins and Matten found that in their trials, participants rapidly lose weight eating a high-sirtfood diet (admittedly, it is calorie-restricted during the first week. More importantly, even without increasing their exercise, they gained muscle mass and showed lower blood sugars and fats.

They also mentioned getting more time, they slept better, they looked better, and they had no hunger problems. Goggins and Matten soon realized that these sirt foods are present in the kitchens of those communities that boast the lowest rate of obesity and disease in the world, most obviously in the Mediterranean diet. It's worth remembering that such items are not rare or unavailable for the most part, and the eating plan is comfortable and practical enough to fit in with every other that you may follow - 5:2, low carb, Paleo, vegetarian, even vegan or gluten-free.

If you choose to follow that diet strictly, you'll need a juicer. You'll drink the green juice three times a day for the first three days, with one meal. Day's 4 to 7 call for two juices and two meals, and you can add just one juice to your standard three meals afterward.

Weight loss of half a stone in the first week is likely, and that includes putting on an average of two pounds of muscle.

Exercise shouldn't be strenuous, though Goggins and Matten suggest that everyone fit for general good health in half an hour a day. The only other recommendation is to seek to avoid eating by 7 pm because calories are absorbed less efficiently by the body as the day goes on.

And, while sirtfoods are plant foods, they also point out that you need to combine them with protein to get full benefits from both. We all know that fried meat should be avoided, and red meat should be kept once or twice a week, but poultry, eggs (and milk in moderation) are excellent, as are lentils and soy, beans, and nuts of course. Sirtfoods do have an especially beneficial omega-3 oils relationship, so include oily fish two to three days a week.

The studies performed by Goggins and Matten at a European health club showed the average dieter losing 7lbs in 7 days and an improvement in muscle mass and general well-being. What exactly is the catch?

Evidence on the health benefits of 'sirtfoods' is still in its early days, and while the diet is perfect for promoting fruit and vegetable intake, if you're hoping for a drastic weight loss, you might be disappointed. Also, the tests conducted on gym members saw participants eat around 1,000 calories for the first three days, then 1,500 for the remaining days, indicating that reducing overall calorie intake and integrating 'sirt foods' into your diet is essential.

1.3 Sirtfood Diet and Weight Loss

While the early phase of juicing and fasting is only suitable for anyone who may want to move a few pounds rapidly, the Sirtfood diet's general approach is to incorporate healthy foods into your diet to improve your well-being and strengthen your immune system throughout time.

Although the first seven days seem tough, the longer-term strategy works for everyone.

By concentrating on incorporating Sirtfood rich ingredients into your everyday meals, you can start burning fat while enjoying usual favorites.

Model Jodie Kidd says, 'People keep asking me my secret to looking great. Aidan's and Glen's Sirtfood diet is the solution. I feel unstoppable since following it. '

Aidan and Lorraine Pascale, TV presenter, said, 'A non-faddy diet that offers incredible health benefits and weight loss. Aidan and Glen show how everyone can reap the benefits of the Sirtfood diet by eating delicious food. I'm a huge fan!'

Ben Ainslie says, 'I'm healthier, more alert, and in top physical condition. Sirtfoods are key for me to reach new peaks in performance to face the upcoming challenges'.

The Sirtfood diet is very restrictive, admittedly. The Sirtfood diet relies primarily on calorie counting as opposed to the Keto or Paleo diets, which stress maintaining a healthy diet. It also requires that you cut to an extreme if only temporarily, certain major food groups and portions downsize. So, you might miss out on lean proteins (beef, chicken, and legumes) for the first week. Although you are also permitted to consume olive oil and walnut (both of these are sources of sirtuin), within the first week, the overall daily calorie intake is incredibly small — less than 50% of what the typical active man wants. Further essential nutrients, such as calcium and iron, are also lacking.

It's still uncertain if sirtuin will help to induce weight loss. To date, no human studies have identified a conclusive correlation between sirtuin-rich foods and weight loss.

Drinking drinks that are rich in vegetables and low in sugar for much of the day will quickly induce short-term weight reduction of their own: if you have fewer calories and remain hydrated, it makes perfect sense to lose a few pounds.

It is backed up by Kristen Smith, MS, RD, LD, a spokeswoman for the Academy of Nutrition and Dietetics. "It is hard to discern if the expected accelerated weight reduction in the first week of diet is due to the extremely low-calorie diet prescribed or linked to the fat-burning properties of sirtuin-boosting foods," she says.

Basically, "regardless of sirtuin-boosting foods, people would lose weight in a 1000-calorie diet," she says.

Alpert's decided. "The authors say people can lose up to 7 pounds in 7 days, but I wonder how much of this weight stays off for more than a month, if so long," she explains.

Even if you lose weight within the first week, it might be mostly water weight, meaning you could get it back once you start taking more calories. In reality, you can even gain weight. As previously mentioned when you lose a lot of weight rapidly, your body's metabolism slows down as your body is trying to compensate for its decreased calorie intake.

Like every diet, it also comes with its side effects. While eating so little in the short term probably won't do much harm, if you're not used to eating so little during the day, it can cause fatigue, nausea, impaired mental focus, and headaches, says Smith. It can also cause unpleasant bowel movements if you don't get enough fiber. What's more, you could get bad breath, a side effect of not eating enough.

Nonetheless, there is one positive: if you consume a lot of sirt foods over a long period, you may find changes in heart health due to polyphenols in foods you eat. If you keep eating sirtfoods after finishing the diet and start consuming more calories, you'll see the benefits.

Undoubtedly the diet tends to work for certain people. Yet scientific evidence of any diet's effectiveness is very different.

Of course, the ideal research to determine the efficacy of a diet on weight loss (or some other result, such as aging) requires a fairly broad sample – representative of the population we are interested in – and random allocation to a treatment or control group.

Results would then be supervised over an appropriate period with strict control over confusing variables, such as other behaviors that may positively or negatively affect interest outcomes, such as smoking or exercise.

This research would be restricted by techniques such as self-reporting and recollection but would go a few other ways to discover this diet's effectiveness.

Nonetheless, work of this type does not exist, and so we should be vigilant when analyzing basic science. After all, human cells in a tissue culture dish possibly respond very differently to a living person's cells.

Further doubt is cast over this diet when considering some specific claims.

Seven-pound losses in one week are unrealistic and very unlikely to reflect changes in body fat.

Dieters consume about 1,000 kcal per day for the first three days – around 40-50% of what most people need.

This will result in rapid glycogen loss (a stored form of carbohydrate) from skeletal muscle and liver.

But we store about 2.7 grams of water for every gram of stored glycogen, and water is heavy.

But we also lose energy for all the glycogen lost - and thus weight.

Furthermore, overly restrictive diets are difficult to obey, resulting in increased appetite-stimulating hormones such as ghrelin.

Thus, weight (glycogen and water) returns to normal if the urge to eat wins.

But thinking of it simply as a weight-loss diet is missing the point. It's a diet that's as much about fitness as waistlines. Increased stamina, clearer skin, more alertness, and improved sleep are the good 'side effects' of this feeding. Often the results are even more surprising, including cases where metabolic disorders have long-term reversed after diet. Such is the health-enhancing effects that studies show them to be more effective than prescription medications to combat cardiovascular illness, with benefits in diabetes, heart disease, and Alzheimer's, to name a few. It's no wonder that the communities consume the most Sirtfoods have become the cleanest and healthiest in the world.

The bottom line is clear: if you want a healthier, leaner, and happier body and lay the foundations for good health and disease resistance, and the Sirtfood Diet is for you.

Remember, it's not a diet. Having 1000kcal for three consecutive days is incredibly difficult, and most people will be unable to achieve it. Looking at the food list, you can see they're the kind of things that always appear on a 'healthy food list,' but it would be easier to promote them as part of a more balanced diet. Occasionally, enjoying a glass of red wine or a small amount of chocolate won't hurt us-but it is not suggested to do it every day. A person on sirtfood diet will eat a mixture of different fruits and vegetables, not just those on the list.

In terms of weight loss and metabolism improving, people may have experienced a seven-pound weight loss on scales, but it would be fluid.

Burning and losing fat takes time, and this weight loss is an incredibly unlikely fat loss. You can be very skeptical about any diet that advocates quick and rapid weight loss because it's just not possible and is more than likely a loss of fluid. When people return to their normal eating habits, they'll regain the weight. The secret to gradual and steady weight loss is to limit calories and increase our activity rates. Eating healthy daily meals with low GI foods, lean protein, fruit, and vegetables, and keeping them well hydrated is the best way to lose weight.

1.4 Effectiveness of Sirtfood Diet

Sirtfoods work by activating the body's so-called "skinny gene" pathways, the same genes activated when exercising or fast.

This makes the body burn fat in a manner that mimics calorie limitation, but without food depletion or other deficiencies.

The sample of people testing the diet, along with increased muscle mass and reports of feeling full and satisfied with food intake, reported an average loss of 7 pounds in 7 days.

There is currently no compelling proof that the Sirtfood Diet has a more positive impact on weight reduction than any other calorie-restricted diet.

And while many of these foods have healthy properties, there have been no long-term human studies to determine if eating a sirt-rich diet has any tangible health benefits.

We have learned that – all calories equal – a diet rich in antioxidants has a drastically different effect on the body than an antioxidant food.

But could you achieve the Sirtfood Diet's outcomes by elevating your vegetable, nut, and omega-3-rich fish consumption? If you can't, it's to be seen.

The Sirtfood Diet is based on dietary (i.e., temporary fix) mentality. That is, a highly restrictive phase 1 follows a less stringent period 2, totaling 21-days. Instead of following a nutrient-dense, antioxidant-rich diet as a way of life, individuals are advised to repeat "whenever you wish for a fat-loss boost."

How many of us gladly entered Restrictive Dieting Land to park at Gallon of Ice Cream Station for three days?

Healthy eating — and weight loss — requires a sustainable, sustainable way to feed your body the nutrients it needs to function optimally, and move.

Sensationalized reports and sometimes hyperbolic portrayal of science evidence add to the nearly relentless debate about whether - and how much - we can consume, increasing our fascination for a 'quick-fix' or miracle remedy, which is itself an entrenched societal crisis.

Many researchers claim that the Sirtfood diet should be consigned to the fad pile for the purposes described - at least scientifically.

Based on the evidence they have, suggesting otherwise is at best spurious and, at worst, misleading and damaging to reasonable public health strategy goals.

The diet is unlikely to support communities facing a diabetes crisis, overshadowed by obesity.

As some have reported very clearly, special diets do not work, and dieting is not a cure for communities where over half of adults are overweight.

Currently, the best strategy is to combine long-term behavioral change with political and environmental influence to increase physical activity and some form of conscious control over what we eat.

It's not a quick fix, but works.

Throughout the 2015 research study (conducted by Goggins and Matten) testing sirtuin efficacy, the 39 participants lost an average of seven pounds in seven days. These results sound impressive, but realizing this is a small sample size studied over a short time is essential. Weight-loss experts also doubt the lofty promises. "The arguments made are very theoretical and extrapolate from research mainly based on basic species (like yeast) at the cellular level. At the cellular level, what happens at the cellular level does not correlate with what happens at the macro level in the human body," says Adrienne Youdim, M.D., Centre for Weight Loss and Diet at Beverly Hills, CA.

Now, the fact that people lose weight following the SirtFood Diet probably results in two main factors:

1. The plan's foods appear to be nutrient-rich.

2. The diet requires you to follow an intense calorie restriction week — 1,000 calories a day for the first three days and 1,500 for the rest of the week. And most of those calories come from the juice.

Limiting calories, as you already recognize, is the most effective weight-loss technique. Interestingly, studies at Finland's Helsinki University showed that low-calorie diets would spontaneously increase sirtuin activity irrespective of whether or not you consume sirtuin-rich foods.

So yeah, introduce some sirtuin foods to your diet: broccoli, bananas, walnuts, buckwheat, celery, red onions — all are nice. If you're concerned about weight reduction, concentrate on lean foods, fruits, and whole grains — and hold reducing the overall calorie consumption.

Researchers investigated the impact of Sirtfoods on safety and weight control. One 2013 study showed that Sirtfood-rich diets tend to assist with safe aging and chronic disease prevention.

A 2017 study found that polyphenols tend to support reducing body weight, blood glucose, and blood pressure — but this field needs further work.

One explanation you'll lose pounds if you adopt the Sirtfood diet right is that you're trying to cut calories (at least in step 1) to 1,000 to 1,500 calories a day, nearly safe drop weight.

The simple truth is that although you don't have to consume sirtuin-activating foods to lose pounds (merely reducing your total calorie consumption will do the trick), most Sirtfoods are safe, tend to lower disease risks and help maintain body weight.

Chapter 2: Benefits and Best Foods of Sirtfood Diet

The Sirtfood Diet promotes healthy food but is restrictive in choices of calories and nourishment. It also involves drinking lots of green juice, which is not a recommendation for regular use.

The Sirtfood diet is low in calories, and not nutritionally balanced in step one. This may leave you hungry, but for the average healthy adult, it is not risky.

It might have some health impacts (positive or negative), which should be considered before starting the diet.

2.1 Sirtfood Diet and its Positive Impact on Health

Sirtfoods include dark chocolate, green tea, and turmeric, which are helpful to the human body. Research, reported in the Clinical Hypertension Journal, showed that high cacao content could reduce the risk of heart disease and help combat inflammation.

The research reported in the journal Molecules showed that turmeric has anti-inflammatory properties and can guard against chronic diseases related to inflammation.

However, before you leap on the fad diet bandwagon, we suggest that you visit a licensed nutritionist because each form of the body is specific, and the dietary needs are different.

While the Sirtfood diet's promise is intriguing (Adele and Pippa Middleton are reportedly fans), and while limiting your calories might cause you to lose weight in the short run, the question remains: is this diet healthy, or is it just another stupid (and potentially dangerous) dietary trend? Is it still thriving in the first place, for that matter?

Sirtfoods are almost always safe options, and they may also provide specific health benefits thanks to their antioxidant or anti-inflammatory effects.

But consuming just a handful of especially nutritious foods cannot serve all the nutritional needs of the body.

The Sirtfood Diet is overly stringent and does not provide any simple, exclusive health benefits over any other diet.

Additionally, consuming just 1,000 calories is not usually advised without a doctor's supervision. For certain men, just consuming 1,500 calories a day is too limiting.

The diet includes up to three green juices a day. Liquids may also be a good source of vitamins and minerals; they are a source of sugar and contain almost none of the nutritious fibers that whole fruits and vegetables do.

What's more, sipping on juice all day is an unfortunate thing for both blood sugar and teeth.

Since the diet is small in calories and food choice, protein, vitamins, and minerals are more than likely insufficient, particularly during the first process.

This diet can be tough to adhere to for the full three weeks owing to the reduced calorie rates and limited food options.

Add this to the high initial expense of needing to purchase a juicer, and certain uncommon and costly products, as well as the time cost of cooking different meals and juices. This lifestyle is unfeasible and impractical for several.

While the Sirtfood Diet's first phase is deficient in calories and nutritionally incomplete, there are no real safety concerns for the average, healthy adult considering the short duration of the diet.

However, calorie restriction and drinking mostly juice for the first few days of the diet can cause dangerous changes in blood sugar levels for someone with diabetes.

Nevertheless, even a safe person can encounter specific side effects — primarily hunger.

Eating just 1,000–1,500 calories a day would leave only about everyone feeling thin, mainly if most of what you're eating is the juice that's low in fiber, a nutrient that makes you feel full.

During step one, you may feel specific side effects such as nausea, lightheadedness, and irritability due to the calorie limit.

Severe health effects are impossible for the normally stable person if the plan is adopted for a mere three weeks.

One great thing about the sirtfood diet is that all the items you will consume on the menu are healthy for you, ensuring the average consumption of vitamins, minerals, and nutrients would be high.

Any diet that will strip out whole food groups may be harmful. It's not very strong research that supports the idea of switching on your skinny gene. The overall Sirtfood diet is very stringent in terms of both food and calories, which may make things challenging to adhere to. There is still little reason to show that weight reduction is a more fruitful approach than any other diet regulated by calories.

The biggest pro is that this diet actively encourages red wine, dark chocolate, and coffee, not something you often hear!

The compounds which make up our favorite treats are abundant in-activators of sirtuin. Though eating a kale smoothie of course accompanied by a whole bar of Green and Blacks does not see you losing the pounds. Anything in balance.

Aiden and Glen claim attendees never feel hunger - which suggests it's perfect for someone who can't get through a regular cleanse day without feeling like they're going to die because they do not have a Huge Mac right away.

A few years back, Sirtfood was a revolutionary food program, which was the favorite lifestyle for the broadsheet papers. The reports say if you skipped it because it contains red wine, candy, and coffee. The response to the issue, 'can you consume meat on the sirt food diet that is much less advertised and attention-grabbing (but still positive news)? 'Yeah, it's a resounding. The diet plan contains a decent quality portion of meat, but it also goes on to say that protein is an integral part of a diet focused on Sirtfood to gain full profit. It's vegetarian-friendly too, so it caters to almost everyone, which is what makes it so good for us an alternative.

There is growing proof that sirtuin activators may have a wide variety of health benefits as well as muscle strengthening and appetite suppression. This involves improving memory, helping the body to regulate blood sugar levels, and cleaning up the harm done by free radical molecules that can grow in cells and contribute to cancer and other conditions.

'Substantial empirical proof exists for the beneficial impact of sirtuin-rich food and drinks consumption in reducing chances of chronic disease,' said Professor Frank Hu, a Harvard University authority on diet and epidemiology, in a recent article in the journal Advances In Diet. A sirtfood food is particularly appropriate as an anti-aging regime.

While activators of sirtuin are present in the plant kingdom, only certain fruits and vegetables have adequate amounts to qualify as sirt foods. Examples include green tea, cocoa powder, and turmeric for the Indian seasoning, spinach, onions, and parsley.

Many of the fruits and vegetables on display in supermarkets, such as tomatoes, avocados, bananas, lettuce, kiwis, carrots, and cucumber, are rather low in-activators of sirtuin. However, that doesn't imply they aren't worth consuming because they have plenty of other advantages.

The benefit of consuming a sirtfood balanced diet is that it's much more versatile than other foods. Simply putting any sirtfoods on top, you might eat right. Or you may be focused on getting them. The 5:2 diet could require more calories on low-calorie days, incorporating sirtfoods to claim.

One surprising result of a sirtfood diet trial is that participants lose substantial weight without sacrificing muscle. Gaining muscle was joint for participants, leading to a more defined and toned look. That is sirtfoods' beauty; they activate fat burning, but they also promote muscle growth, maintenance, and repair. This is in direct comparison to other diets where weight reduction usually occurs from both fat and muscle, with muscle loss slowing down the metabolism and finding it more challenging to lose weight.

2.2 Who Shouldn't Follow Sirtfood Diet?

The nutritionists wouldn't recommend a sirtfood diet with diabetes. Because it is extremely important for a diabetic person to consume food at specific times because they lose control over their hunger. When you go ahead in the first stage of this program, you can expect side effects like headaches or lightheadedness as the body adapts to lower calorie intake.

So clearly, it's not recommended for pregnant or conceiving women.

Plan's first week is pretty extensive and tough. Days one to three are highest with your calorie intake restricted to 1000 - combined with three juices and one dinner.

Days four to seven are lenient with a maximum of 1,500 calories per day.

Although this can cause weight loss in the short term, the Sirtfood diet is ultimately so restrictive that it isn't sustainable. So if you've ever had an eating disorder or problematic eating relationship in the past, it's best to stop it entirely.

Three reasons to take a sirtfood diet pass:

1. Sirtfood diet only measures weight loss success.

As said earlier, and it is going to come again: weight is a health determinant, but not the only one. Measuring someone's health performance on how they lose X pounds in X period excludes all other nutritional benefits. Food is full of strength to do things like showering, exercising, and breathing. This also has nutrients that can facilitate several bodily functions and is also a happy tradition-based experience. Focusing on good wellbeing is so much more than just appearance, so assessing performance only in terms of weight loss is incomprehensive.

2. It's restrictive, which can harm your food relationship.

This diet promotes a daily intake of 1,000 to 1,500 calories, far lower than most people need. When we drastically restrict our food intake, our instinctive response is overeating. Your body is smart, considering this lack of sustenance as an attack. So we tend to overcompensate, which is why we can all relate to being "hangry"(hungry and angry), and therefore overindulging when we finally get a chance to eat. Practicing cautious and intuitive eating is healthier than limiting food.

3. The diet is not science-based.

While there is some controversial research on sirtuins' benefits, there is little to no research on the specific sirt food diet. We do have several standards that have been thoroughly studied and tested for decades.

If you're confused about what "good food" is, it's a great place to start.

If you want to add a few sirtfoods into an eating schedule, it's perfect. Foods like green tea, nuts, dark chocolate, and kale all have a balanced eating plan! But adhering to these strict pass-or-fail criteria is impractical and may be detrimental to your food relationship. By implementing a variety-filled eating plan and eating carefully, you will be able to build a long-term, healthy food relationship. Cheers, that!

The diet is very restrictive and less healthy than Keto or Paleo. It focuses on calorie counting and involves cutting large food classes. You'll need to downsize your parts, particularly in week one. Another downside is the lack of essential nutrients like calcium and iron.

If your food intake is not restricted during the day, you may also experience nausea, dizziness, difficulty concentrating, fatigue, and headaches.

However, the 'Sirtfood Diet' is generally best avoided for someone who has dealt with eating disorders in the past or has difficulty regimenting portion control.

If you've already had an unhealthy relationship with food or complicated eating disorder in the past, it's wise to ignore hopping on the Sirtfood Diet Wagon. Instead, add more of the Sirtfoods as mentioned earlier to your diet and cut out processed foods and sugar.

There is no specific category of people who are strictly restricted to follow this diet. But we know our bodies better and understand their demand.

2.3 Top 20 Best Foods Included In Sirtfood Diet

The diet includes a collection of the top 20 foods rich in sirtuins, which seems more like a compilation of popular foods than a complicated new diet. Examples include arugula, chilies, chocolate, green tea, dates of Medjool, red wine, turmeric, walnuts, and even health-conscious kale. Some doctors suggested that although the food is being marketed as safe, it does not automatically encourage weight reduction.

Some of the items that make this a dignified news lifestyle were wine and dark chocolate. All these foods have a place in our diet because their high levels of antioxidants can help protect us against certain chronic diseases and cancers.

The Sirtfood diet's real purpose is to load up one's meals with as many "sirtuin-activating nutrients" as practicable. Sirtuin genes have been activated in laboratory settings. Still, it is noted that despite a pilot study by Goggins and Matten, which analyzed 40 people on a diet, no other studies had been conducted in humans.

"Sirtfoods are all readily available, and plant foods free," Goggins said. "Some of the best Sirtfoods contain arugula, kale, and parsley, almonds, walnuts, olive oil extra virgin, dark chocolate, curry spices, green tea, red wine, and coffee."

On a diet, Goggins and Matten recommend trying to "sirtify" meals where possible and adding Sirtfoods to favorite meals or replacing natural ingredients with an alternative Sirtfood.

Nutritionist has lauded the diet's food options but said there's little to prove the diet's foods can activate the genes as marketed.

They suggest that they don't know if these particular foods can cause such stuff if you consume only certain items, and nothing else.

These are the top 20 Sirtfood diet foods and how you should integrate them into your everyday meals.

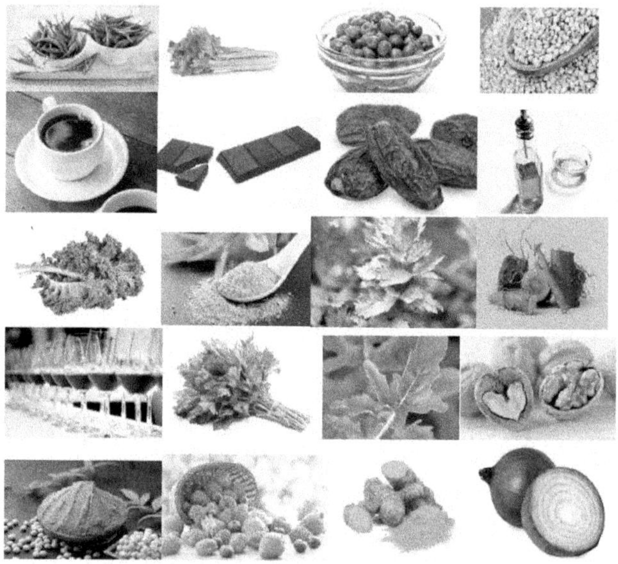

1. Bird's eye chili. Often sells as Thai chilies, and they're more active than standard chilies and more nutrient-packed. Use them to start sweet or sour recipes.

2. Celery. The most valuable component is the heart and the seeds, but don't turn them out if you mix a shakeup.

3. Capers. They are pickled flower buds in case you're curious. Sprinkle over salad or cauliflower toast.

4. Buckwheat. Technically a pseudo-grain: in fact, it is a rhubarb-related fruit seed. Also available in noodle shape (as soba), but be sure to get the wheat-free version.

5. Coffee. Drink it dark-there is some proof that milk can enhance sirtuin-activating nutrient absorption.

6. Cocoa. The type high in flavonol increases blood pressure, regulation of blood sugar, and cholesterol. Check for a large portion of cacao.

7. Medjool dates. They are a massive 66 percent sugar, but they don't raise blood sugar levels in moderation and have been linked to lower diabetes and heart disease rates.

8. Extra virgin olive oil. The additional virgin form has more Sirt advantages and a flavor that is more pleasing and peppery.

9. Kale. It contains large quantities of quercetin and kaempferol, nutrients that trigger sirtuin. To use as salad, soak it with lemon juice and olive oil.

10. Green tea or matcha. Add one slice of lemon to increase sirtuin-producing nutrient absorption. Matcha is even better, but to avoid potential contamination with lead, go to Japanese, not Chinese.

11. Lovage - An herb. On a windowsill, please create your own, and turn it into stir-fries.

12. Chicory. Red is the strongest, but yellow does fit well. Place a bowl over it.

13. Red wine. You've heard of resveratrol: the good news is, its heat stable, so you can take advantage of cooking with it (as well as directly glugging it). Pinot noir has the maximum content.

14. Parsley. Rather than a garnish – it's rich in apigenin. Put it to the full value of a smoothie or tea.

15. Arugula - Rocket. One of the least interfered-with available salad greens. Season with olive oil.

16. Walnuts. Rich in calories and fat but well known to minimize metabolic disease. Smash them to a sirt-flavored pesto of parsley.

17. Soybeans and miso are highly in-activators of sirtuins. Have these in stir-fries.

18. Strawberries and Blueberries. While they are delicious, they produce just 1/100 g of sugar, so evidence shows that they boost the body's capacity to absorb sugar carbohydrates.

19. Red onion. The red kind is excellent for you, so it's good enough for raw food. Chop it and add to a sandwich, or have a burger with it.

20. Turmeric. Data indicates that turmeric has anti-cancer effects in it. Assimilating it alone is unpleasant for the body, but boiling it in liquid and incorporating fat and black pepper improves absorption.

Chapter 3: Getting Started with Sirtfood Diet

In this swift setting, where no one appears to have room for planned meals, meal preparation does not seem a priority. Still, it is precisely because of our quick lives, and our little time to take care of our well-being that meal planning falls into practice, making sure we remain as safe and comfortable as possible. For starters, if you want to alleviate the burden of worrying about what to prepare next, mainly if you do it for a big family, with hard eaters or people with dietary restrictions, meal planning certainly would change your life.

If you start a new diet, it's advised to do it the way it's done to achieve the desired result without making adjustments.

To meet the prescribed recommendations, the sirtfood diet requires the same dedication and rigor.

Let's explore this chapter to get a thorough understanding of the phases of the sirtfood diet and how to begin the diet.

3.1 Understanding the Phases of Sirtfood Diet

The Sirtfood diet seeks to achieve the same impact as exercise and fasting by controlling the calorie consumption and avoiding items that have a number of sirtuin proteins in them (a.k.a. "sirt products").

The Sirtfood Diet is split down into two stages. The first process, which lasts three days, is the hyper-success process which allows you to restrict your daily calorie intake by consuming three green juices and one sirtfood-rich meal a day to 1000 calories a day (You raise your meal count from day's 4 to 7 to two meals and two green juices a day). It is a 7-day regimen that has been shown to successfully lose 7lbs.

On day's four to seven, calorie consumption rises to 1,500 calories, consisting of two green juices rich in Sirtfood and two meals rich in Sirtfood.

The second phase, the "maintenance" process, lasts 14 days and allows you to consume three sirtuin-rich meals and one green juice a day. Phase 2 is a recovery period where weight reduction begins gradually. It's more about packing the diet full of an abundance of Sirtfoods that is accomplished by consuming three nutritious Sirtfood-rich meals a day, along with a Sirtfood green juice for 'maintenance.'

The juices contain spinach, celery, rocket, parsley, lemon, and green tea. Meals contain turkey escalope with buckwheat noodles, basil, capers and parsley, chicken and kale curry, and prawn stir-fry.

The sirtfood diet will cause the activation of certain proteins called sirtuins or colloquially nicknamed skinny genes which have several roles and are a community of seven proteins contained in the body that have been shown to control a number of functions, including digestion, inflammation, and lifespan.

Although the diet encourages healthier foods, it is restrictive, particularly during the initial phases, with both the food preferences and regular calories. It also includes consuming water, with the recommended quantities meeting the existing average requirements during both phases.

In the second phase of the 14 day recovery period, you will witness that there is a gradual weight loss. The pioneers of this diet think it's a practical and safe way to lose weight. Focusing on weight loss, however, is not what the diet is about – it's designed to be about eating the best food that nature has to offer.

They recommend three balanced sirtfood-rich meals a day along with one sirtfood-green juice over the long term too.

This means that you can continue the same group of foods even after you have finished both the phases of diet because it is healthy otherwise, too.

When you think about following a diet, the first thought is some tasteless and plain meals, but with garlic, chicken, and kale curry and prawn stir-fry with buckwheat noodles or sesame-glazed tofu, the meal might be something like turkey escalope. Even if you are vegetarian, you can enjoy delicious recipes made purely from the list of sirtfood. Everything is made up of ingredients rich in Sirtfood.

If you have a sweet tooth, you can also get 15-20 g of dark chocolate after your meal.

The focus shifts to eating 'normally' again after the initial stage of fasting, but upping your intake of the healthy Sirtfoods.

You can go back to the 2 nd chapter's unit 2.3 to read the list of top 20 foods again.

3.2 How to Start the Diet-The best mode to follow

The best mode to follow any diet is to follow it as it is suggested. When you mix your own ingredients in a recipe or mess up with the measurements as suggested by a recipe, you end messing the whole dish. Similarly, if you add your own ideas in a suggested diet, you can never achieve the results claimed by it.

That's why the best mode to follow any diet plan is to follow it as is without customizing it.

The sirtfood diet is a kind of diet that requires a serious commitment in the first week to get desires results. If you don't follow it correctly, you may end up wasting your time.

Week 1- On a Sirtfood diet, you restrict your calorie consumption to 1,000 calories a day and consume three green Sirtfood juices a day. Sirtfood green juice ingredients include kale, arugula, parsley, celery, including leaves, half a green apple, half a lemon juice, and matcha green tea. You may have it over ice or add water but don't include plant-based milk or any other ingredients not mentioned above.

Week 2. You can increase calories to 1,500 a day and consume just two of the Sirtfood Juices a day, and eat two sirtfood meals a day. Carry with this path once you have gained the optimal amount of weight your body requires to feel the greatest.

The safe, gradual, and consistent weight reduction would add up. If you drop 2 or 3 pounds a week, this ensures you'll have gained 15 pounds in five weeks. Bear in mind this Adele weight didn't disappear immediately. The weight loss became noticeable by the end of 2019, and if you've got more than a modest sum or drop, remind yourself that patience is the secret to holding things moving.

There is a nutrition program during both the phases that are not based on calories but on small servings, well-balanced meals, and loading up on mainly sirt products. The 14-day maintenance schedule involves three dinners, one green juice, and one or two treats of sirtfood bits. Followers are encouraged to complete 30 minutes of activity five days a week per recommendation, but it is not the plan's primary focus.

Regular juices are essential to the Sirtfood Diet. And make sure you've got a juicer there. You'll need three main ingredients too.

Matcha is a green tea paste and an essential component in natural juices. It is freely accessible online if it is not kept at the nearest health food shop.

Similarly, lovage - a herb in the recipe for green juice - may also appear impossible to obtain. But purchasing seeds online is simple for growing them in a pot on a windowsill.

Buckwheat, at the end. It's a great alternative to more traditional grains, but most supermarkets in their goods combine buckwheat and wheat. You are more likely to find buckwheat products in your local health food store at 100 percent.

Try soy yogurt with mixed berries, chopped walnuts, and dark chocolate for breakfast, or an omelet packed with bacon, red chicory, and parsley for something savory.

The sirtfood salad is excellent for lunch-but if you want some carbs, a whole meal pitta with turkey, cheese or hummus is healthy and filling.

Stir-fried prawns with kale and buckwheat noodles are a great evening meal too. Whether it's rendered the sirtfood route, believe it or not, pizza is always on the line.

There are approximately 20 different foods that can be classified as sirt foods (as discussed in 2.3). These include kale, red wine, strawberries, ointment, soy, parsley, green tea matcha, buckwheat, turmeric, walnuts, coffee, etc.

The eating schedule is tailored to a weekly timetable.

There's no fixed schedule to execute after those three weeks of diet are finished. All you have to do to start on the Sirtfood route is to change each of your meals to contain as many Sirtfoods as possible. Exercise is often promoted (30 minutes physical activity, five days a week), but feeling sweaty isn't the weight-loss plan's fundamental purpose.

When you are done with both phases of diet, you are done with the diet program.

After that, it is up to you to reboot the phases. That is where the nutritional guidelines tended to become ambiguous because they don't provide a clear timetable of how many occasions such steps will be replicated. The lack of guidance here makes some nutritionists nervous because there may be some long-term implications of repetitive caloric restriction, which we have discussed in previous chapters.

3.3 A Sample Meal Plan

First of all, meal prep involves making a well-planned food schedule by choosing the correct recipes. Do not only use a random selection of ingredients, but work about them, a couple of days sooner than what you want to continue, make it simpler to plan a grocery list, buy, and then really cook the dishes.

You will continue with step 1 when you adopt the Sirtfood diet – which lasts for seven days. As discussed previously, you must consume three Sirtfood drinks during the first three days of the diet, then have one Sirtfood-rich meal for a minimum of 1,000 calories a day. You will consume 1,500 total calories on days four through seven, drink two green juices, and eat two healthy Sirtfood-rich meals. Step 1 is complete.

Phase 2 lasts for 14 days, requiring you to consume three nutritious Sirtfood-rich meals and one green juice a day. You will follow a more rational way of eating after Phase 2 is complete—but are encouraged to include sirtuin-activating foods in regular meal plans. Any time you decide to shed additional weight or body fat, you will re-enter steps 1 and 2.

Keeping these concepts in view, here is what, during the maintenance process, might be on the menu over a week (green juices aside).

There are plenty of breakfast, lunch, and dinner choices open, like:

Breakfast:

- Omelet with Kale
- Muesli, blueberries and yogurt
- Fruit smoothie made with soy milk and dried oats

Lunch & Dinner:

- Fish, tomato and cucumber rocket salad covered in olive oil
- Stir fry, vegetable-packed spicy tofu with bird-eye chili
- Buckwheat-grilled tuna with salad or pasta salad
- Stir-fried with chicken and soba noodle
- Tofu burgers with salad and wholegrain bread
- Kale salad in olive oil with edamame beans and red onion
- Spicy chicken curry eaten with brown rice in wholegrain

Snacking:

- Coffee
- Hummus and celery
- Fresh fruit, particularly strawberries and apples and oranges
- Pasta
- Dark chocolate bar

Throughout the last chapter are given some fantastic recipes for breakfast, lunch, and dinner.

Now let's talk about a sample plan. Below is a sample diet plan for your ease, you can customize the meal options as per your choice:

Phase 1 consists of two distinct stages:

Day 1 to Day 3: These are the most critical and the most serious. You will eat up to a maximum of 1,000 calories per day during this period. It consists of:

- 3 servings Stirfood green juices (recipe issued at the end of the unit)
- 1 serving of the main meal

Day 4 to Day 7:

You can raise your calorie consumption to a maximum of 1500 calories per day in these days:

- 2 serving of Sirtfood green juices
- 2 servings of main meals

7-Day Schedule:

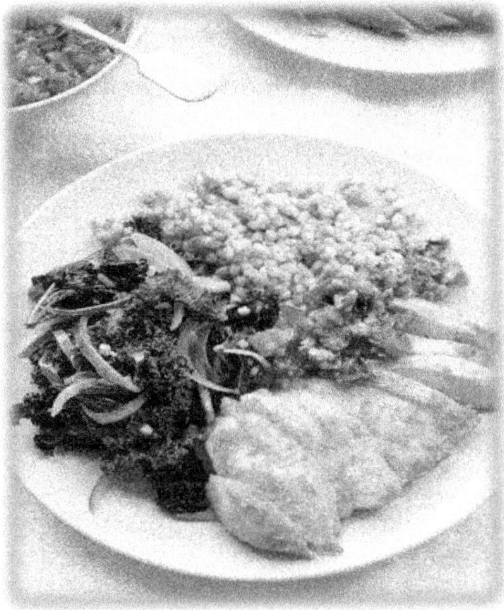

Work on a Seven Day Plan to make Step 1 effective.

Let's begin each day with a thorough plan:

Monday:

Breakfast:

A glass of Sirt juice before or after breakfast with 2 tiny bits of protein, including one hard-boiled egg white and 1 3 oz. piece of chicken.

Lunch/Dinner:

Any main meal from the sirtfood diet recipes (turmeric chicken and kale salad with honey-lime dressing) with a glass of Sirt juice.

Snack:

A handful of walnut or a small 85 percent dark chocolate and tea/coffee.

Evening:

1 glass of Sirt juice.

Drink lots of water for the whole day and try to limit meal consumption before 7 pm in the evening.

Tuesday:

Breakfast:

A glass of Sirt juice before or after breakfast with 2 tiny bits of protein, including one hard-boiled egg white and 1 3 oz. piece of chicken.

Lunch/Dinner:

Any main meal from the sirtfood diet recipes (Tuscan bean stew) with a glass of Sirt juice.

Snack:

Fresh fruits (strawberry, apple, and oranges) or a small 85 percent dark chocolate and tea/coffee.

Evening:

1 glass of Sirt juice.

Drink lots of water for the whole day and try to limit meal consumption before 7 pm in the evening.

Wednesday:

Breakfast:

A glass of Sirt juice before or after breakfast with 2 tiny bits of protein, including one hard-boiled egg white and 1 3 oz. piece of chicken.

Lunch/Dinner:

Any main meal from the sirtfood diet recipes (Oriental salmon and broccoli tray bake) with a glass of Sirt juice.

Snack:

6 oz. red wine a small 85 percent dark chocolate and tea/coffee

Evening:

1 glass of Sirt juice.

Drink lots of water for the whole day and try to limit meal consumption before 7 pm in the evening.

Thursday:

Breakfast:

A glass of Sirt juice before or after breakfast with 3 bits of protein with hard-boiled egg white or other breakfast meal and 1 3 oz. piece of chicken/other meat.

Lunch:

Any main meal from the sirtfood diet recipes (Coronation chicken salad) with a glass of Sirt juice.

Snack:

6 oz. red wine a small 85 percent dark chocolate and tea/coffee.

Dinner:

Any main meal from the sirtfood diet recipes (Asian king prawn stir-fry with buckwheat noodles)

Drink lots of water for the whole day and try to limit meal consumption before 7 pm in the evening.

Friday:

Breakfast:

A glass of Sirt juice before or after breakfast with 3 bits of protein with hard-boiled egg white or other breakfast meal and 1 3 oz. piece of chicken/other meat.

Lunch:

Any main meal from the sirtfood diet recipes (Aromatic chicken breast with kale and red onion and tomato with chili salsa) with a glass of Sirt juice.

Snack:

6 oz. red wine a small 85 percent dark chocolate and tea/coffee.

Dinner:

Any main meal from the sirtfood diet recipes (Strawberry buckwheat tabouleh)

Drink lots of water for the whole day and try to limit meal consumption before 7 pm in the evening.

Saturday:

Breakfast:

A glass of Sirt juice before or after breakfast with 3 bits of protein with hard-boiled egg white or other breakfast meal and 1 3 oz. piece of chicken/other meat.

Lunch:

Any main meal from the sirtfood diet recipes (Fragrant Asian Hotpot) with a glass of Sirt juice.

Snack:

6 oz. red wine a small 85 percent dark chocolate and tea/coffee.

Dinner:

Any main meal from the sirtfood diet recipes (Baked Potato with spicy chickpea stew)

Drink lots of water for the whole day and try to limit meal consumption before 7 pm in the evening.

Sunday:

Breakfast:

A glass of Sirt juice before or after breakfast with 3 bits of protein with hard-boiled egg white or other breakfast meal and 1 3 oz. piece of chicken/other meat.

Lunch:

Any main meal from the sirtfood diet recipes (Kale and red onion dhal with buckwheat) with a glass of Sirt juice.

Snack:

6 oz. red wine a small 85 percent dark chocolate and tea/coffee.

Dinner:

Any main meal from the sirtfood diet recipes (Miso marinated cod with stir-fried greens and sesame)

Drink lots of water for the whole day and try to limit meal consumption before 7 pm in the evening.

After completing the first phase successfully, it's time to move on to the next step that is phase 2 – the maintenance phase.

This is a 14-day period. With a healthy breakfast, you'll be moving to a more natural schedule with three meals a day.

It can be the sirtfood smoothie, sirt muesli, or some other breakfast meal, as mentioned in this book's last chapter.

Start your morning with a healthy sirt breakfast after three meals per day and have your green juice first thing. It's perfect for waiting a couple of hours before getting breakfast because after drinking a glass of green juice, a lot of people feel complete. Yet don't overpower it.

Alternatively, you may resume your day with a decent meal and then wait for the green juice for two or three hours. Do whatever you like.

What about the snacks?

You could have snacks. Even if you implement the meal plan as mentioned above, there's not enough space for snacking.

14-Day Schedule:

Every day you will get the following in this 14-day meal plan:

- 1 serving of Sirtfood juice.
- 3 main meals.
- Up to 2 snacks on sirtfood.

The juice should be consumed in the morning as a first item, or at least 30 minutes until eating.

Day1-Day 14

A ton of water, tea/coffee, 1 serving of Sirt juice once a day (3 bits of protein with hard-boiled egg white and 1 3 oz. piece of chicken/any meat), a tiny square of dark chocolate two times a day or assorted treats twice a day, lunch and dinner with an extra meal - recipes from the last book.

Recipe for Sirtfood Green Juice:

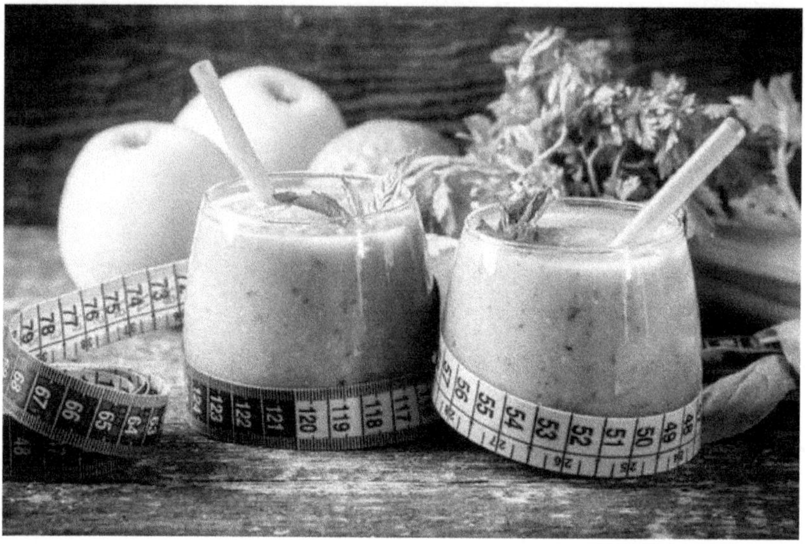

Serves 1

Appliance required: A juicer

Ingredients:

- 2 Large handfuls (2.5 oz.) of kale
- A large pinch (1 oz.) of arugula
- Quite a low pinch (1/4 oz.) of parsley with flat leaves
- 2 to 3 full (5.5 oz.) stalks of celery with leaves
- 1/2 Mild Apple Gray
- New ginger, 1/2- to 1-inch
- 1/2 Lemon Juice
- 1/2 Level Matcha Teaspoon Powder

Directions:

Blend the kale, arugula, and parsley, juice them—next, the celery, apple, and ginger juice. Squeeze lemon into the juice. Put some juice into a glass, add matcha, mix and wait before it dissolves. Add remaining juice, add a stirring finish, drink or top with plain water.

3.4 Organize Your Diet Schedule

Organizing your diet is really important to be consistent in the schedule and be prepared for the days of your diet so that you may not leave it in the middle due to any lacking resources.

Some general tips are discussed below to organize your diet schedule:

1. Start with Modest Goals: it can appear daunting to look at weight maps. Looking at a goal is necessary, but it begins low. People normally concentrate only on exercising more as they began searching for a balanced diet schedule. Afterward, they start consuming more vegetables or diet food. They don't drop a lot of weight, but they would feel healthier and appeared excellent.

2. Make step by step reduction targets for weight. Do not rush into losing weight. Hold things off by consuming more nutritious meals rather than having fewer meals. When you think you are ready to start the diet, go for it.

3. Holding good health is the priority: Everyone love looking healthy and receiving congratulations, but the greatest encouragement is ensuring that you will be able to live longer and safer and keep up with your family. For this, you need to have a healthy diet instead of a strict diet, which omits all the necessary food out of your diet.

You need to know: To operate on a balanced diet plan:

- Number of servings of each form of food you need every day.
- Part measurements right.

Few Suggestions on sample sizes:

Measure or measure all of your food for a week, or before you can accurately determine one part.

Use tiny plates and bowls. If it fills up your little bowl or dish, it will make you see a serving as "full."

Each day using the same pot or pan. Try to consider having the same bowl you're your muesli or salad makes calculating portion size convenient for you.

Buy plates display separated part sizes portions proper. These plates are perfect for everyone, but especially beneficial if you want to teach children how to eat the right quantities.

Take one part of the meal you'll have on the pan, and then go out for seconds if you're still hungry. You often want to pile up on more food when you're hungry, but if you just take one serving size to eat first, you will find it is enough. However, if you put on two servings, you would always consume all of that only because it's on your plate!

Think about the leftovers-a couple of days later, they are instrumental. Choosing recipes that last you longer means you don't have to cook every day, and you can repurpose the main elements in various combinations.

Mix the fresh and the familiar. Always have a collection of recipes you learn with all your heart, and your family enjoys; those you can eat over and over again.

Spend some time preparing the dream meal. Often it can feel that a recipe takes so long to produce, but generally, it's worth it if you can't wait to try it but cannot find the right time.

You are your friend to that, easy, and nutritious ingredients. Think of what you already have in the kitchen and continue from there. This is the fastest and fastest way to get going. And you avoid wasting food as well as spending any extra money, which is a very beneficial effect of any healthy meal plan.

4. Plan forwards, but not too far ahead. Shopping and organizing fit well in most situations and for most individuals about a week in advance, but there are several variations, of course. It is essential to still bear in mind how many meals you are going to eat at home before you schedule your next meal and shopping trip. Before entering the grocery store, it is essential to know precisely what you want to buy, even when shopping every day.

5. Shop first from the refrigerator and closets of the pantry. Don't ignore any single thing you already have in the refrigerator, freezer, or cupboard - you want to save some time and make use of the products that you still have at home. Create your meal plan based on which food is going to waste faster, then add the rest of the ingredients to your list. You will keep control of your diet by holding a chart of inventories at hand. This means you won't miss the extra food that is waiting deep in the freezer for you.

6. Stay rid of anything that is not worthy of the current meal schedule. The best way is to get rid of everything else that's not on the menu plan you've just completed or listed in the table of healthier choices. Anything that has to go.

7. Now you're going to have to crack old habits because even if you've de-cluttered your kitchen because pantry and refrigerator, those old habits are already rooted in your home in both significant and tiny ways. Look at the food that is still in your fridge and pantry again. Be honest—does it all refer to the existence we try to build for you in those spaces? You need to restart. Old customs die hard. It is time they were purged for good. Here you are at a critical turning stage. Plunge into the deep end. Engage or not-your call.

8. Take your calendar out and prepare meals that match the schedule of the week

Here are several items to remember when you pick the recipes and create a plan:

- What would you do in advance? Could you replicate all of those recipes?
- How would you crockpot for meetings or extracurricular events for active evenings?
- When to effectively exploit the leftovers? (Some recipes speak about it too!)
- Don't skip your balanced lunch and breakfast products!

9. Prepare meals for you.

Below are a few more suggestions for rising duplication and make the preparations perfect:

- Take a couple of extra measures before putting away your grocery to transform your nutritious choices into fast food! Rubbery dry carrots?! Wash and cut fruit and veggies for snacking, and put them in the fridge at eye level.
- Attach any notes you'll like for the week to your schedule - take the meat out or place it in the daily crockpot.
- Have unused portion for lunch.

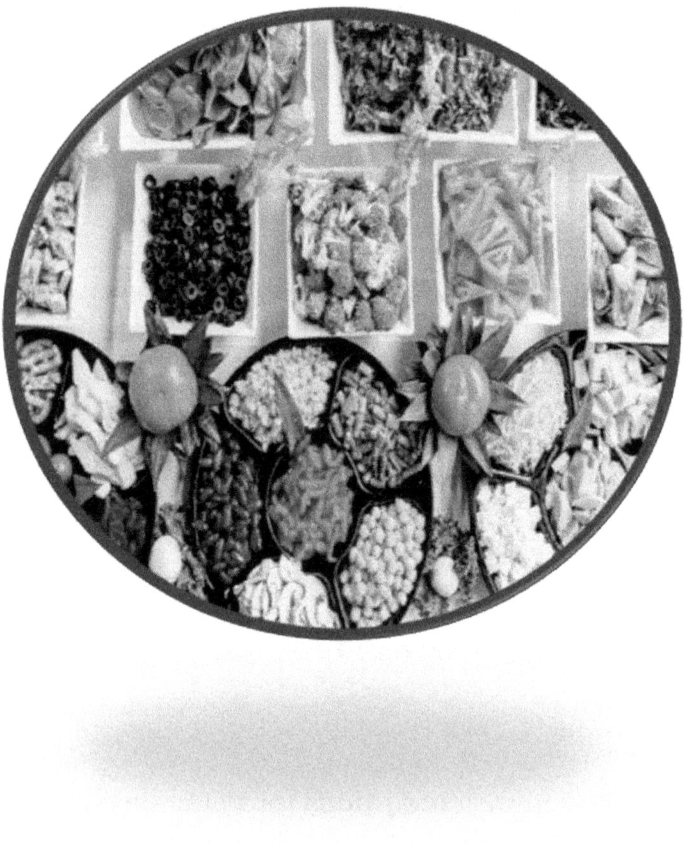

Chapter 4: Factors to Consider while Following the Diet

If it comes to weight management, it is widely accepted that the safest way is to implement balanced dietary habits along with physical exercise to offset energy consumption against calorie production, rather than adopting fad diets.

However, as the number of overweight and obese people in the US and around the world is growing, many nutritional approaches and resources are surfacing, including diets focused on protein, meal replacement foods, non-prescription food drugs, and much more.

Here we'll address all the things you need to remember before, during, and after the sirtfood diet program.

4.1 Sirtfood Diet VS. Other Diets

Sirtfoods are indeed compliant with all other nutritional strategies but also significantly improve their wellbeing and weight gains substantially. This applies to diets currently very popular such as intermittent fasting, low-carb, paleo, and gluten-free diets. Eating a portion of food rich in Sirtfoods means that intermittent fasting's calorie restriction can be less severe, yet the benefits will be the same if not higher. A 7-day advantage, rather than just saying five on the 5:2 day fasting scheme.

The addition of Sirtfoods will significantly improve low-carb diets that lack plant-based foods. The overwhelming majority of Sirtfoods Top 20 are small in carbohydrates.

Sirtfoods are archetypal paleo products, including the sirtuin-activating polyphenols consumed by humans and reaping the rewards of countless years before. Sirtfoods is a piece of paleo philosophy that is missing.

To give a clearer picture and understand different types of diet, let's have a look at some of the other popular diet plans.

<u>1,200 Diet Calorie:</u>

As the name suggests, the intake limit for this diet is 1,200 calories per day.

The U.S. Dietary Guidelines recommend an intake of between 1,600 to 2,400 calories per day for adult women, and 2,000 to 3,000 calories per day for men.

Lauri Y. Wright, Ph.D., an adjunct professor of public health at the University of North Florida, says cutting calories is essential for those who want to lose weight.

The key to weight loss is to create a calorie deficit. The system then relies on accumulated fat for the necessary energy of the body, which is seen as weight loss, as explained by Wright. We take care of diets that are very limited as deficient calorie diets will permanently slow down the metabolism. Very small is usually known to be below 1,200 calories for women and 1,500 calories for men.

It is essential that those calorie-restricting ones still meet their nutrient needs.

As per the view of Wright, the diet must contain all the necessary nutrients that are important to wellness. The smaller the calories, the easier it will be to provide all the required nutrients, vitamins, and minerals. It is suggested to consult a licensed dietitian who can prepare the healthiest meal habits to meet the health objectives.

Dana Hunnes, Ph.D., a senior dietitian at the University of California Los Angeles Medical Center, says that cutting calories to 1200 a day is not sustainable in the long term unless a person has low-calorie needs or is under the direct guidance of a medical professional.

Unlike a long-term dietary plan, this will probably be called a crash diet, so it is not really suggested by Dana. It's best to lose weight slowly over time, and in a manner that's manageable throughout life, this is not that eating strategy because it's not enough. It'd slow down your metabolism because it'd not be enough calories.

Fasting intermittently:

Intermittent eating was one of the leading diet-search words for 2019.

Kristin Kirkpatrick, a licensed dietitian, and health nutritional services manager at the Cleveland Clinic Health Center of Ohio explains that there are two major variations of the most simple terms: Time-limited feeding (TRE), which is consuming strictly over an 8-hour to 10-hour span, to a 5:2 solution where people consume just 500 calories divided into two meals, two days a week. Men get 600.

According to her, the effects are vast, including healthy life, weight reduction, and decreased likelihood of cardiovascular illness.

Hunnes says other possible positive effects of intermittent fasting include benefits to the gastrointestinal system by giving it time to rest and decrease inflammation in the body. But it isn't suitable for everybody that quick.

Wright argues that intermittent fasting isn't a safe idea for pregnant people or those with other disorders of health, including diabetes. One research showed that intermittent fasting might affect cardiac wellbeing. Additionally, the body may recover weight quicker after losing weight with intermittent fasting as the body perceived fasting as deprivation.

No Fat, No Carbs:

Singer Jennifer Lopez announced earlier this year that she was trying a 10-day challenge, with no carbohydrates and no sugar. Lopez invited her fans to enter her a few days into her diet.

Experts claim, however, that some carbs are required.

According to Hunnes, our brains rely on carbohydrate-derived glucose for safe functioning, much like our muscles do. This form of diet is not safe. Of course, it is good to reduce or eliminate sugar, not to restrict all carbohydrates.

Wright concurred that carbohydrates are important to wellbeing. Furthermore, the issue for certain citizens is the amount and volume of carbohydrates eaten. This is essential to consider complex carbohydrates such as whole-grain portions of pasta, rice, beans, vegetables, and berries, rather than simple sugars such as soda and sweets.

Wright added that apart from the energy required to fuel the body, carbohydrates also provide important vitamins, minerals, and fiber. Carbs are necessary and cannot be omitted from the diet. Rather, select balanced carbs and monitor quantities. Excessive carbohydrates will create unnecessary calories and trigger elevated diabetic blood sugars.

Wright suggests that an appropriate portion of carbohydrate would behalf to one cup of pasta instead of a whole plate, or one-third to two-thirds of a cup of rice, rather than an entire bowl.

Ultra Keto Diet:

Last year, one of Google's leading food results was the high weight, low carb Keto Diet.

This year, a diet variation called "Keto Ultra," which includes supplements, has made the top 10 diets most sought after.

About this diet, Wright explains that the ketogenic diet is deficient in carbs and very heavy in sugar, placing the body in ketosis — fat oxidation in place of food glucose. The Keto diet has been seen to minimize weight, and like any diet that limits whole food groups, decreased dietary diversity may lead to lower calorie consumption. A side effect of ketosis is decreased appetite, which often leads to weight loss.

Although the diet has threats to it.

Thanks to the absence of carbohydrate-containing products such as fruits, berries, whole grains, and beans, a ketogenic diet may lead to some vitamin and mineral shortages and can have a detrimental effect on the wellbeing of the stomach according to Wright. The reduction of muscle mass has also been reported to people on a ketogenic diet, which is especially troublesome for older adults.

Hunnes insists that a keto-based diet is not safe.

He says that he doesn't believe that it is a good option because evolutionarily speaking, we are dependent on carbohydrates as our main source of nutrition. A high-fat, high-protein diet isn't safe for us at all. He does not suggest a ketogenic diet in the best possible words.

Both Wright and Hunnes mention that the only individuals who may profit from a keto-based diet are infants having epilepsy and adopting the plan with their doctor's professional advice.

In babies and adolescents under professional observation, the ketogenic diet has been shown to control serious epilepsy effectively.

4.2 After-Effects of Sirtfood Diet

If you adopt the diet strictly, you will lose weight. If you eat 1,000 calories of tacos, 1,000 calories of kale, or 1,000 calories of snicker doodles, you're going to lose weight at 1,000 calories! Yet it is also noted that, with a more rational calorie limit, you will have results. The average regular calorie consumption of those not on a diet is between 2,000 and 2,200, but reducing to 1,500 is still limiting and should be a successful weight-loss plan for most people,

This strategy is strict with no wiggle room or substitutions, so weight control will only be achieved if the reduced calorie consumption is still sustained, rendering long-term commitment impossible. That ensures that any weight you lose in the first seven days after you stop, is likely to be gained back. Its main concern? Limiting the intake of protein with juices will result in a loss of muscle mass. Losing muscle is synonymous with dropping your metabolic rate or 'metabolism,' making it harder to maintain weight.

There are other ways you can decrease your calorie intake without being so restrictive in the food you eat. That being said, the diet isn't actually "unhealthy," and if a person experienced improvement, he wouldn't automatically be wary about it.

If you implement this strategy, make sure to consume lots of nutrients and change the food you eat to prevent shortages in vitamins. The diet is incredibly strict and has not been adequately proven to be effective. You are much better off developing a lifestyle in the proportions that suit your individual needs to eat a variety of whole foods.

After finding that a small group may replicate the effects of fasting and exercise by triggering sirtuin in the body, it was pilot-tested by writers Aidan Goggins and Glen Matten and found that the participants lost an average of 3.18 kg in 7 days while retaining or even raising their muscle mass.

The viability of this program, in the long run, is uncertain. After you've been through the first few weeks, there's no dietary plan to adopt except to attach more Sirtfoods to each meal. This makes the diet far more flexible than most, which is a huge advantage, but a three-week-long stretch of deprivation could easily lead to overeating during phase two, ultimately putting you back on square one.

This is always a stressful lifestyle to adopt, even though you're uber-disciplined. Some doctors state that many people would feel starving for a mere 1,000 calories. And if you're not a green juice addict, a first week favorite, it will make you much thirstier. Also, since most of the phase one weight loss is water weight, it will come back on once you resume healthy eating.

Moreover, following any diet that does not include a healthy amount of protein (e.g., the Sirtfood diet's first week), muscle loss and slower metabolism may result. Creating muscle by consuming lots of nutrition and exercising with weights is essential for weight reduction and holding it off.

In addition to all this, work on SIRT-1 inducing foods is still very much in its infancy, and it is uncertain if eating polyphenol-rich foods would have a significant effect on weight in general. Weight is a multi-faceted concept that involves complex interactions between our unique genetic makeup and diet, patterns of movement, sleeping habits, and emotional state.

Ultimately, consuming a diet high in a range of nutritious ingredients, including lean protein products, different fruits and vegetables, and whole grains, is a safer, natural way to lose weight and hold it off.

Although its proponents say it's not a fad diet, health professionals caution that the Sirtfood diet might not be conducive to weight reduction because it's not nutritionally healthy. The food is also deficient in calories, which isn't a healthy way to do that.

Eating just 1,000-1,500 calories a day can leave you feeling starving. In the first step, you may even feel other side effects such as lightheadedness, nausea due to intense calorie cutting. So, the Sirtfood Diet isn't a healthy, sustainable plan, though a rapid weight loss strategy may not be a bad idea. You would also contact a doctor or dietitian before carrying out the Sirtfood Diet schedule, along with in all other diet plans.

The bottom line is, the healthiest and easiest way to build and sustain a healthy mind and body is to get a proper diet paired with daily exercise.

All-in-all, from the naked eye, the Sirtfood diet doesn't look that poor. But it does have a few significant gripes for the dietitians.

To continue with, at the beginning of step one, some of its opponents are not a fan of the intense restriction. The idea that this phase detoxifies your body seems vague to them. They argue that your organs are more than capable of doing that.

Moreover, living on a mere 1000 calories a day is really hard work. Incessant pangs of hunger are excruciating, not to mention the effect on the social life it might have. During this process, you probably won't be able to fulfill your regular nutrient needs, either, due to the overall food shortages. There are drawbacks of extended fasting, of course, but that is not for all.

Another factor they wouldn't suggest it is the mere fact that this is a 'diet.' The strict rules on food can be too challenging to adhere to - and you'll actually give in, feel bad, and then resume the diet again, and keep making that loop to never really get anywhere.

It also grinds the gears when diets like this place those items on a pedestal as though it's a silver cure-all product should and should be part of a balanced diet, it's true. What's essential is diversity, rather than eating a few select foods in large amounts.

You would generally understand the severe complexity before trying to follow the 'Sirtfood Diet,' which has already been reported by dietitians. Considering that it limits carbohydrates, it is mostly geared towards weight loss in the short term, so if you're looking to sustain weight loss, a different diet or eating plan may be more manageable in the long run.

The writers argue that the Sirt diet's target is more about balanced eating than about drastic weight loss. However, some nutritionists have taken offense to the fact that their aim is decorated with the tag line "lose 7lbs in 7 days" A reduction of 1 to 2lbs a week is seen as a stable and balanced number. And in a brief amount of time, such drastic weight reduction may not be ideal for your health. Again, visible but relevant: red wine is full of contaminants, even though it is rich in sirtuin activators, so it certainly isn't a smart idea to guzzle it as part of a 'diet.'

4.3 When to Stop the Diet?

With 52 percent of Americans confessing that they consider it harder to pay their taxes than learning how to eat healthily, adopting a method of eating that is a way of life rather than a one-off fad diet is essential.

It might not be too challenging for us to lose weight or maintain a healthier weight, but the Sirtfood diet may support those dealing with it. Yet what about mixing the Sirtfood diet with exercise, is it advisable to entirely skip a workout or incorporate exercise after you have begun the diet?

With an estimated 650 million obese adults worldwide, finding healthy eating and exercise regimes that are doable is essential, not depriving you of everything you enjoy, and not requiring you to exercise all week. That is precisely what the Sirtfood diet does.

The theory is that such foods stimulate the receptors of the 'skinny gene,' which are usually triggered by fasting and exercise. The good thing is, some food and beverages, including dark chocolate and red wine, contain chemical substances called polyphenols that activate the genes that mimic the effects of exercise and fasting.

It should be wise to avoid or increased exercise during the first week or two of the diet where the calorie consumption is limited as the body adapts to fewer calories. Listen to your body and don't work out if you feel tired, or have less energy than usual. Instead, make sure you remain focused on the concepts that contribute to a balanced lifestyle, such as having sufficient dietary food, calcium, and fruit and vegetable rates. It's essential to consume protein, ideally one hour after your workout, when doing exercise.

During the workout, protein strengthens the body, decreases soreness, and may aid regeneration. Several recipes contain protein that would be ideal for consumption after a workout, such as sirt chili con carne or turmeric chicken and kale salad. You might try the sirt blueberry smoothie if you want anything lighter and add some protein powder for added value. You will be down to the type of fitness you do, but home workouts will allow you to choose when to exercise, the types of exercises that suit you, and are short and convenient.

The diet of Sirtfood is a perfect way to improve your dietary patterns, lose weight, and feel healthier. You may be challenged by the initial few weeks, but it's essential to check which foods are best to eat and which delicious recipes are right for you. Over the first few weeks, be kind to yourself as your body adapts and take exercise quickly if you want to do it at all. If you are already somebody who does moderate or intense workout, you may be able to carry on as usual or manage your fitness in line with the dietary change. As with any changes in diet and exercise, the whole thing is about the individual and how far you can push yourself.

This is based on a strict plan that includes calorie control-1000 for the first three days, then up to 1500-and consumes a set number of green juices and Sirtfood-rich meals. But the aim is to eat as many Sirtfoods as possible in the long term.

The Sirtfood Diet Plan Side Effects & Precautions:

One may feel hungry while following this diet due to low-calorie intake. Consultation with the doctor is advised before following some diet. The results vary from person to person, depending on the body's need. Persons with lipid disorders, diabetes, lung failure, and hormonal imbalances should be prevented.

So we can conclude that there is no fixed time to stop the diet. You have to listen to your guts. Whenever you feel like you cannot take it anymore, you should stop it right away.

Chapter 5: Sirtfood Diet Recipes without Compromising Taste

You want to talk about starting the sirtfood diet, and for that, you have to get some perfect recipes in hand for all occasions.

Whether it's an office dinner, a date-night for a pair, family meals, or just fulfilling your appetite, we've got you covered with some fantastic sirtfood recipes to ease your appetite and hold you on a diet.

5.1 Meals for Office

Below are some snack ideas and lunch meal recipes for your workplace.

Snack Ideas

Choc Chip Granola:

Ingredients:

- 200g jumbo oats
- 2 tbsp. rice malt syrup
- 3 tbsp. light olive oil
- 20g butter
- 50g pecans, chopped

- 60g good-quality (70%) dark chocolate chips
- 1 tbsp. dark brown sugar

Directions:

- Oven preheats to 160°C (140°C fan / Gas 3). Cover a large baking tray with parchment of silicone or baking.
- In a wide pot, add the oats and pecans. Steam the olive oil, butter, brown sugar, and rice malt syrup gently in a medium non-stick pan before the butter has melted and the sugar and syrup have dissolved. Do not let simmer. Pour the syrup over the oats and mix vigorously until completely coated with the oats.
- Scatter the granola over the baking tray and distribute it out through the corners. Leave the mixture clumps with mixing, instead of just scattering. Bake for 20 minutes in the oven until the sides are tinged light brown. Remove from the oven, and allow absolutely to cool on the plate.
- Once it is cold, smash with your fingertips any larger lumps on the tray and add in the chocolate chips. Place the granola in an airtight container or pot, or spill it. The granola is to last for at least two weeks.

Date & Walnut Cinnamon Bites

INGREDIENTS:

- 3 walnut halves
- 3 pitted Medjool dates
- the ground cinnamon, to taste

DIRECTIONS:

- Cut each walnut carefully into three slices, and do the same with dates. Put a slice of walnut, brush with cinnamon, and serve.

Lunch

Sesame Chicken Salad

Ingredients:

1 tbsp. sesame seeds

150g cooked chicken, shredded

100g baby kale, chopped

60g pak choi, finely shredded

½ red onion, finely sliced

Large handful (20g) parsley, chopped

1 Cucumber, peeled, half-long, deseed with a tablespoon, sliced

For the dressing:

1 tbsp. extra virgin olive oil

1 tsp. sesame oil

Juice of 1 lime

1 tsp. clear honey

2 tsps. soy sauce

Directions:

In a dry saucepan, roast the sesame seeds for 2 minutes until lightly browned and fragrant. Switch to cool board.

Blend the olive oil, sesame oil, lime juice, honey, and soy sauce together in a tiny bowl to create a dressing.

In a wide pot, put the cucumber, the kale, the pak choi, the red onion, and the parsley and combine gently. Pour over the sauce, once again combine.

Spread the salad with the grilled chicken between two sides, on top. Shortly before eating, brush over the sesame seeds.

Braised Puy Lentils

Ingredients:

8 Cherry tomatoes halved

2 tsp. Extra virgin olive oil

40 g Carrots, peeled and thinly sliced

40 g Red onion, thinly sliced

1 Garlic clove, finely chopped

40 g Celery, thinly sliced

1 tsp. Thyme (dry or fresh)

1 tsp. Paprika

50 g Kale, roughly chopped

75 g Puy lentils

220 ml Vegetable stock

20 g Rocket

1 tbsp. Parsley, chopped

Directions:

Heat oven 120°C / gas 1/2.

Roast the tomatoes in a small roasting tin for 35–45 minutes.

Heat a casserole over low-medium heat. Apply 1 teaspoon of olive oil with red onion, garlic, celery, carrot, and fry for 1–2 minutes until smooth. Add paprika and thyme and cook for another minute.

Wash the lentils in a fine-meshed sieve and add them to the stock. Bring to boil, may heat, and cook gently for 20 minutes with a lid on the oven. Stir the pot every 7 minutes or so, adding water if it falls too far.

Add kale and cook for 10 minutes. When baked, stir in the parsley and roasted tomatoes. Serve with the rocket with the remaining olive oil tablespoon.

Turmeric Chicken with Kale Salad and Honey Lime Dressing

Ingredients:

For the chicken

½ medium brown onion, diced

1 teaspoon ghee/1 tbsp. coconut oil

1teaspoon lime zest

½ teaspoon salt + pepper

1 large garlic clove, finely diced

1 teaspoon turmeric powder

1teaspoon lime zest

250-300 g / 9 oz. chicken mince or diced up chicken thighs

juice of ½ lime

For the salad

½ avocado, sliced

2 tablespoons pumpkin seeds (pepitas)

a handful of fresh parsley leaves, chopped

3 large kale leaves, chopped without stems

a handful of fresh parsley leaves, chopped

6 broccoli stalks/2 cups of broccoli florets

a handful of fresh coriander leaves, chopped

½ avocado, sliced

For the dressing

3 tablespoons lime juice

3 tablespoons extra-virgin olive oil (you can use 1 tablespoon avocado oil and 2 tablespoons EVO)

1 garlic clove, finely chopped or grated

1 teaspoon raw honey

½ teaspoon wholegrain or Dijon mustard

½ teaspoon sea salt and pepper

Directions:

Over the medium to high heat, cook the ghee or coconut oil in a small saucepan. Attach the onion and sauté for 4-5 minutes, until golden. Add thin chicken and garlic and stir 2-3 minutes over medium-high heat, breaking apart.

Add the lime zest, lime juice, turmeric, salt, and pepper and cook for another 3-4 minutes. Set aside the thin fried.

While cooking, put a small saucepan of water to boil. Add broccoli, cook 2 minutes. Rinse under cold water, cut into 3-4 bits.

Attach the pumpkin seeds from chicken and toast over medium heat for 2 minutes, always stirring to avoid burning. Season with some water. Set aside. Pure pumpkin seeds are also useful.

Place kale in a salad bowl and pour over the dressing. Toss and mix the kale with the dressing. This will soften the kale, like what citrus juice does to Carpaccio fish or beef - it's slightly cooking.

Finally, shake the cooked rice, broccoli, fresh herbs, pumpkin seeds, and avocado slices.

Strawberry, Tomato & Watercress Salad with Honey & Pink Pepper Dressing

INGREDIENT:

300g strawberries

250g mixed tomatoes

100g watercress, woody stalks discarded

1 tbsp. pink peppercorns

2 strawberries (about 40g), chopped

½ tbsp. honey

½ lemon, juiced

3 tbsp. extra virgin olive oil

DIRECTIONS:

Toast the peppercorns in a dry saucepan for 1-2 minutes until fragrant, then bash quickly with a pestle and mortar to crack the skins. Add the 2 strawberries and paste them.

Remove honey and lemon juice. Put the dressing in a large bowl and whisk in oil. Check for seasoning, add salt or lemon juice if you prefer. Break the strawberries into quarters or thin wedges and cut the tomatoes finely, slicing some and halving others, so you get plenty of different shapes. Mix the bowl's watercress.

Divide the salad into four plates or onto a pan. Spoon over some bowl-left dressing.

Red Chicory, Pear & Hazelnut Salad

Ingredients:

2 heads of red, or white if not available

2 ripe red Williams pears

a good handful of rocket leaves

25g hazelnuts toasted and chopped

For the dressing

2 tbsp. hazelnut

2 tbsp. any mild salad oil, such as sunflower oil/safflower oil/olive oil

1 tsp. sherry or cider vinegar

1 tsp. green peppercorns in brine, optional

Directions:

Make dressing. Using green peppercorns, gently smash them in a wooden spoon tub, or use a pestle and mortar. Mix the oils and vinegar with salt.

Trim the chicory stalk and remove any dead or tired outer leaves. Separate the leaves carefully and arrange 5-6 on 4 plates, if large, cut or break into pieces.

Remove the stalks and quarter the pears lengthwise. Cut stems, slice the fruit thinly. Arrange the pear slices over the chicory leaves and spoon half the dressing.

Pour over the remaining dressing, season with salt and pepper.

Give the leaves a short toss on each salad. Sprinkle with nuts, drink.

Buckwheat Pasta Salad

Ingredients:

50g buckwheat pasta(cooked)

large handful of rocket

1/2 avocado, diced

8 cherry tomatoes, halved

20g pine nuts

a small handful of basil leaves

10 olives

1 tbsp. extra virgin olive oil

Directions:

Mix all the ingredients, except for the pine nuts, gently and place on a dish or in a bowl, then spread the nuts over the edges.

5.2 Delicious Recipes for Couples

Breakfast

Smoked Salmon Omelet

Ingredients:

2 Medium eggs

100 g Smoked salmon, sliced

1/2 tsp. Capers

10 g Rocket, chopped

1 tsp. Parsley, chopped

1 tsp. Extra virgin olive oil

Directions:

Whisk the eggs finely in a bowl.

Add the salmon, capers, parsley, and shot.

In a non-stick frying pan, fire up the olive oil until heated but not burning.

Remove the egg mixture and transfer the mixture across the plate.

Use a spatula or fish slice until it is even.

Reduce flame and let cook through the omelet.

Slide the spatula along the sides and roll the omelet up or split in half to eat.

Kale and Blackcurrant Smoothie

Ingredients:

2 tsp. honey

1 cup freshly made green tea

10 baby kale leaves, stalks removed

1 ripe banana

40 g blackcurrants, washed and stalks removed

6 ice cubes

Directions:

Add the honey into the moist green tea until it dissolves. Whiz all of the ingredients in a blender together until creamy. Serve straight away.

Date and Walnut Porridge

Ingredients:

200 ml Milk or dairy-free alternative

1 Medjool date, chopped

35 g Buckwheat flakes

1 tsp. Walnut butter or 4 chopped walnut halves

50 g Strawberries, hulled

Directions:

Place the milk and date in a casserole, heat gently, cook the buckwheat flakes until the porridge is the perfect consistency.

Add walnut butter or walnuts, cover with strawberries, and eat.

The Sirtfood Diet's Shakshuka

Ingredients:

1 tsp. extra virgin olive oil

40 g Red onion, finely chopped

1 Garlic clove, finely chopped

30 g Celery, finely chopped

1 Bird's eye chili, finely chopped

30 g Kale, roughly chopped without stems

1 tsp. Ground cumin

1 tsp. Paprika

1 tsp. Ground turmeric

400 g Tinned chopped tomatoes

1 tbsp. Chopped parsley

2 Medium eggs

Directions:

Heat a small, deep-sided pot over medium-low heat. Add oil and fry for 1–2 minutes onion, garlic, celery, chili, and spices.

Add tomatoes, then leave the sauce to cook for 20 minutes, stirring occasionally.

Add kale and cook another 5 minutes. If the sauce is too deep, easily add more water.

Stir in parsley when your sauce has a right, creamy consistency.

Create two little sauce wells and smash growing egg into them.

Cover with a cap or foil and lower the heat to low.

Leave the eggs to cook for 10–12 minutes, where the whites should be firm while the yolks are still runny.

Cook another 3–4 minutes if you prefer firm eggs. Serve immediately – ideally straight.

Lunch

Buckwheat Noodles and Chicken Kale with Miso Dressing

Ingredients:

For the noodles

3-4 shiitake mushrooms, sliced

2-3 handfuls of kale leaves (removed from the stem and roughly cut)

150 g / 5 oz. buckwheat noodles (100% buckwheat, no wheat)

1 brown onion, finely diced

1 teaspoon coconut oil or ghee

1 long red chili, thinly sliced (seeds in or out depending on how hot you like it)

1 medium free-range chicken breast, sliced or diced

2-3 tablespoons Tamari sauce (gluten-free soy sauce)

2 large garlic cloves, finely diced

For the miso dressing

1½ tablespoon fresh organic miso

1 tablespoon Tamari sauce

1 tablespoon extra-virgin olive oil

1 tablespoon lemon or lime juice

1 teaspoon sesame oil (optional)

Directions:

Take a small saucepan with boiling water. Add the kale and cook until mildly wilted, for 1 minute. Remove and put aside, then carry the water back to the boil. Add the noodles and cook (usually around 5 minutes) according to package directions. Place apart and rinse under the cool spray.

While, in a little ghee or coconut oil (about a teaspoon), pan fry the shiitake mushrooms for 2-3 minutes, until well browned on either side. Sprinkle with salt from the sea, then put back.

Heat more coconut oil or ghee in the same frying pan over medium to high heat. Stir in onion and chili for 2-3 minutes, then incorporate pieces of meat. Cook over medium heat for 5 minutes, stirring a few times, then add the garlic, tamari sauce, and some splash of water. Cook for another 2-3 minutes, always stirring before the chicken is cooked through.

Finally, introduce the kale and soba noodles and cook up by swirling through the food.

At the end of the preparation, blend the miso dressing and drizzle over the noodles to hold all the helpful probiotics alive and working in the miso.

Asian King Prawn Stir-Fry and Buckwheat Noodles

Ingredients:

75g soba (buckwheat noodles)

2 tsp. extra virgin olive oil

2 tsp. tamari (You can also use soy sauce without gluten.)

150g shelled raw king prawns, deveined

1 garlic clove, finely chopped

1 bird's eye chili, finely chopped

1 tsp. finely chopped fresh ginger

20g red onions, sliced

40g celery, trimmed and sliced

75g green beans, chopped

50g kale, roughly chopped

100ml chicken stock

5g lovage or celery leaves

Directions:

Steam a frying pan over high fire, then cook the prawns 2–3 minutes in 1 teaspoon tamari and 1 teaspoon oil. Transferring prawns to a tray. Wipe the kitchen paper pan clean before you need it again.

Cook the noodles for 5–8 minutes or as indicated on the box. Drain, put aside.

In the remaining liquid, fry the garlic, chili, and ginger, red onion, celery, beans, and kale over medium-high heat for 2–3 minutes.

Add stock and bring to simmer, then cook for a minute or two until the vegetables are cooked but crunchy.

Add the prawns, noodles, and leaves of lovage/celery to the plate, carry back to simmer, remove from heat, and drink.

Italian kale

INGREDIENTS:

3 tbsp. olive oil

3 garlic cloves, finely sliced

3 tbsp. red wine vinegar

300g cavolo nero or kale, roughly shredded

DIRECTIONS:

Let the oil heat up in a wide pan with a lid, heat the garlic, and then add some vinegar and tea.

Tip the kale into the oven, cover in the steam for 4-5 minutes, adding more water if the oven becomes too warm. When wilted, season with a pinch of sea salt.

Tuscan Bean Stew

Ingredients:

1 tbsp. extra virgin olive oil

50g red onion, finely chopped

30g carrot, peeled and finely chopped

30g celery, trimmed and finely chopped

1 garlic clove, finely chopped

½ bird's eye chili, finely chopped (optional)

1 tsp. herbes de Provence

200ml vegetable stock

1 x 400g tin chopped Italian tomatoes

1 tsp. tomato purée

200g tinned mixed beans

50g kale, roughly chopped

1 tbsp. roughly chopped parsley

40g buckwheat

Directions:

Place the oil over low-medium heat in a medium saucepan and fry the onion, carrot, celery, garlic, chili, if used, and herbs until the onion is soft but not cooked.

Remove stock, tomatoes, and purée and bring to boil.

Remove beans and cook 30 minutes.

Add the kale and cook for another 5–10 minutes, then introduce the parsley.

Meanwhile, after the package directions, cook the buckwheat, rinse and serve with the stew.

Dinner

Super healthy salmon salad

INGREDIENTS:

100g couscous

1 tbsp. olive oil

200g sprouting broccoli, roughly shredded without larger stalks

juice 1 lemon

2 salmon fillets

a small handful of pumpkin seeds

seeds from half a pomegranate

olive oil and some extra lemon wedges, to serve

2 handfuls watercress

DIRECTIONS:

In a steamer, heat the water.

Season the couscous with 1 tsp. butter.

Pour boiling water over the couscous, cover 1 cm, then set aside. After heating the water in the steamer, tip the broccoli into the broth, then place the salmon in the tier above.

Process before salmon is ready and broccoli soft.

Drain broccoli and cool under the cold spray.

Combine remaining oil and lemon juice—cast broccoli, pomegranate seeds, and pumpkin seeds into the lemon dressing couscous.

At the last second, cut the watercress and throw it into the couscous.

Serve with salmon, lemon wedges, and fresh olive oil to drizzle, if you prefer.

Malabar prawns

INGREDIENTS:

400g raw king prawns

2 tsp. turmeric

3-4 tsp. Kashmiri chili powder

4 tsp. lemon juice, plus a squeeze

40g ginger, half peeled and grated, half finely sliced into matchsticks

1 tbsp. vegetable oil

4 curry leaves

2-4 green chilies, halved and deseeded

1 onion, finely sliced

1 tsp. cracked black pepper

40g fresh coconut, grated

½ small bunch coriander leaves only

DIRECTIONS:

Rinse in cool water and pat warm.

Connect the turmeric, chili powder, lemon juice, and grated ginger and put aside.

Steam oil in a saucepan and incorporate curry leaves, pepper, sliced ginger, and onion.

Cook for about 10 minutes, then apply the black pepper.

Stir-fry the prawns with some marinade until fried, around 2 minutes.

Season if necessary, add lemon juice squeeze. Serve with coconut and coriander leaves.

Chicken, Beetroot and Broccoli Salad with Avocado Pesto

Ingredients:

250g thin-stemmed broccoli

100g bag watercress

2 tsp. rapeseed oil

1 red onion, thinly sliced

3 skinless chicken breasts

1 tsp. nigella seeds

2 Fresh beetroots (about 175 g), peeled and sliced

For the avocado pesto

½ garlic cloves, crushed

small pack basil

25g walnut halves, crumbled

1 avocado

1 tbsp. rapeseed oil

juice and zest 1 lemon

Directions:

Bring a wide pan of water to simmer, add broccoli, and cook 2 minutes.

Drain, rinse under the cool spray.

Warm a griddle plate, swirl the broccoli in 1/2 tsp. of the rapeseed oil and skillet for 2-3 minutes, rotating until slightly charred.

Set aside cool.

Clean the chicken with oil and season—grid for 3-4 minutes each side or before cooking. Nice, slice or cut into chunky bits.

And render pesto.

Pick the basil leaves and set aside a few to finish the salad.

Place the remainder in a food processor's cup.

Scoop avocado flesh and add cloves, walnuts, butter, 1 tbsp. lemon juice, 2-3 tbsp. cold water and some seasoning to the food processor.

Blitz until flat, switch to a serving bowl. Pour over the sliced onions and quit for a few minutes.

Place watercress on a large pan.

Toss broccoli and onion with the lemon juice they were washed in. Cover with beetroot, just don't combine it with food.

Scatter over-retained basil berries, lemon zest, and nigella beans, then top with pesto avocado.

Prawn Arrabbiata

Ingredients:

Raw or cooked prawns (Ideally king prawns)

65 g Buckwheat pasta

1 tbsp. Extra virgin olive oil

40 g Red onion, finely chopped

1 Garlic clove, finely chopped

30 g Celery, finely chopped

1 Bird's eye chili, finely chopped

1 tsp. Dried mixed herbs

1 tsp. Extra virgin olive oil

2 tbsp. White wine (optional)

400 g Tinned chopped tomatoes

1 tbsp. Chopped parsley

Directions:

Fry onion, garlic, celery, and chili in the oil over medium-low heat for 1–2 minutes.

Switch heat to normal, add the wine, and cook 1 minute.

If the sauce is too deep, Remove the tomatoes and allow the sauce to simmer over medium-low heat for 20-30 minutes until right, rich consistency.

Easily add more water.

While preparing, carry a pan of water to the boil and cook the pasta as instructed by the packet. Drain, mix with the olive oil and hold in the pan until desired.

Add the raw prawns to the sauce and simmer for another 3–4 minutes before they become pink and opaque, attach the parsley, and eat.

When using fried prawns, add the parsley, put the sauce to the boil, and eat.

Attach the cooked pasta, combine thoroughly yet softly, and eat.

5.3 Treat Yourself with Easy Recipes -Recipes for Singles

Breakfast

Sirt Fruit Salad

Ingredients:

½ cup freshly made green tea

1 tsp. honey

1 orange, halved

1 apple, cored and roughly chopped

10 red seedless grapes

10 blueberries

Directions:

Pour over half a cup of green tea. When dissolved, add half-the-orange juice. Leave nice.

Split the other half of the orange into a bowl with the sliced tomato, grapes, and blueberries.

Pour over the cooled tea and brew a few minutes before eating.

Sirt Muesli

Ingredients:

20g buckwheat flakes

10g buckwheat puffs

15g coconut flakes or desiccated coconut

40g Medjool dates, pitted and chopped

15g walnuts, chopped

10g cocoa nibs

100g strawberries, hulled and chopped

100g plain Greek yogurt (or vegan alternative, such as soya or coconut yogurt)

Directions:

Mix all the above items together (leave strawberries and milk if not eaten immediately).

<u>Raspberry and Blackcurrant Jelly</u>

Ingredients:

100g raspberries washed

2 leaves gelatin

100g blackcurrants washed and stalks removed

2 tbsp. granulated sugar

300ml water

Directions:

Place raspberries in two dishes/glasses/molds. Placed gelatin leaves in the cold water bowl to soften.

Put the blackcurrants in a small sugar and 100ml water pan and bring it to a boil. Simmer vigorously for 5 minutes, remove from oil. Let stay for 2 minutes.

Extract excess water from gelatin leaves and add to saucepan. Drain when drained, then drain the remaining vapor. **Load the liquid onto the dishes and refrigerate.**

Jellies will be available in 3-4 hours or overnight.

<u>Grape and Melon Juice</u>

Ingredients:

Half cucumber, sliced if desired, cut and finely minced.

100 g cantaloupe melon, sliced, split into chunks

100g red seedless grapes

30g young spinach leaves stalk removed

Directions:

Mix together in a juicer or blender until smooth

Lunch

Sirt Food Miso Marinated Cod with Stir-Fried Greens & Sesame

Ingredients:

20g miso

1 tbsp. mirin

1 tbsp. extra virgin olive oil

200g skinless cod fillet

20g red onion, sliced

40g celery, sliced

1 garlic clove, finely chopped

1 bird's eye chili, finely chopped

1 tsp. finely chopped fresh ginger

60g green beans

50g kale, roughly chopped

1 tsp. sesame seeds

5g parsley, roughly chopped

1 tbsp. tamari

30g buckwheat

1 tsp. ground turmeric

Directions:

Mix miso, mirin, and oil 1 tablespoon. Rub over the cod and marinate for 30 minutes. Temperature up to 220oC / gas 7.

Bake cod 10 minutes.

Heat a large saucepan or wok with remaining oil. Stir-fry the onion for a few minutes, then incorporate the celery, garlic, pepper, ginger, green beans, and kale. Toss and fry until soft and cooked clean. You may need to add some water to the pan to help cook.

Cook the buckwheat for 3 minutes according to the package directions.

Attach stir-fry sesame seeds, parsley, and tamari and serve with greens and shrimp.

Kale and Red Onion Dhal with Buckwheat

Ingredients

1 tablespoon olive oil

1 small red onion, sliced

2 teaspoons turmeric

3 garlic cloves, grated or crushed

2 cm ginger, grated

1 bird's eye chili, deseeded and finely chopped (you can add more if you like it hot!)

400ml coconut milk

160g buckwheat (or brown rice)

2 teaspoons garam masala

160g red lentils

100g kale (or spinach would also be a great alternative)

200ml water

Directions:

Put the oil in a big, deep saucepan and add the sliced onion. Cook on low heat for 5 minutes until softened.

Add garlic, ginger, chili and simmer for 1 minute.

Add turmeric, garam masala, splash water, and cook for 1 minute.

Add red lentils, coconut milk and 200ml water (simply fill the coconut milk with water and pour into the saucepan).

Mix it properly and cook over a gentle heat for 20 minutes. Stir regularly and apply water if the dhal starts to adhere.

After 20 minutes, introduce the kale, vigorously mix and remove the cap, cook for another 5 minutes (1-2 minutes if you use spinach instead!)

Place buckwheat in a medium saucepan about 15 minutes until curry is ready and add plenty of boiling water. Carry the water back to the boil and simmer for 10 minutes (or longer if you want softer buckwheat. Drain the buckwheat and serve with the dhal.

Coronation Chicken Salad

Ingredients:

75 g Natural yogurt

1 tsp. Ground turmeric

Juice of 1/4 of a lemon

1 tsp. Coriander, chopped

100 g grilled chicken breast, bite-sized pieces

1/2 tsp. Mild curry powder

1 Medjool date, finely chopped

6 Walnut halves, finely chopped

20 g Red onion, diced

1 Bird's eye chili

40 g Rocket, to serve

Directions:

Layer milk, lemon juice, coriander, and spices in a mug. Serve the remaining components on a rocket pad.

Broccoli and Green Kale Soup

INGREDIENTS:

500ml stock, / in a jug of boiling water add 1 tbsp. of bouillon powder

1 tbsp. sunflower oil

2 garlic cloves, sliced

thumb-sized piece ginger, sliced

½ tsp. ground coriander

3cm/1 slice of fresh turmeric, peeled and dried, or 1/2 tsp of turmeric powder

pinch of pink Himalayan salt

200g courgettes, roughly sliced

85g broccoli

100g kale, chopped

1 lime, zested and juiced

small pack parsley, roughly chopped, reserving a few whole leaves to serve

Directions:

Put the oil in a deep pan, add the garlic, ginger, coriander, turmeric and salt, fry on medium heat for 2 minutes, and then apply 3 tbsps. of water to the spices.

Add the courgettes, making sure you blend properly to cover all the spices, and finish cooking for 3 minutes. Connect 400ml stock and cook 3 minutes.

Add broccoli, kale and lime juice with the remaining stock. Cook another 3-4 minutes before all vegetables are tender.

Drop fire and apply chopped parsley. Load all into a mixer, combine until smooth at high rpm. It should be a pretty leaf with dark-colored parts (which is the kale).

Garnish with lime and parsley.

Dinner

<u>Strawberry Buckwheat Tabouleh</u>

Ingredients:

50g buckwheat

1 tbsp. ground turmeric

80g avocado

65g tomato

20g red onion

25g Medjool dates pitted

1 tbsp. capers

30g parsley

100g strawberries, hulled

1 tbsp. extra virgin olive oil

juice of ½ lemon

30g rocket

Directions:

Cook buckwheat with turmeric as per package instructions.

Drain and cool to one side.

Chop the mango, basil, red onion, almonds, capers, and parsley and blend with the buckwheat.

Cut the strawberries and softly blend oil and lemon juice in the salad.

Serve on the rocket board.

Baked Salmon Salad Topped With Creamy Mint Dressing

Ingredients:

1 salmon fillet (130g)

40g mixed salad leaves

40g young spinach leaves

2 radishes, trimmed and thinly sliced

5cm piece (50g) cucumber, cut into chunks

2 spring onions, trimmed and sliced

1 small handful (10g) parsley, roughly chopped

For the dressing:

1 top low-fat mayonnaise

1 tbsp. natural yogurt

1 tbsp. rice vinegar

2 leaves mint, finely chopped

Salt and freshly ground black pepper

Directions:

Let the oven preheat to 200°C (180°C fan / Gas 6).

Growing the salmon fillet on a baking tray and bake for 16–18 minutes until cooked. Remove from the oven, put aside.

The salmon is hot or cold in the salad. If your salmon has meat, quickly separate the salmon from the meat using a fish slice after frying. Easily slip off when fried.

Blend mayonnaise, mustard, rice wine vinegar, mint leaves, salt, and pepper in a medium bowl and allow to stand for at least 5 minutes.

Placed on a serving plate lettuce leaves and spinach and finish with radishes, cucumber, spring onions, and parsley. Flake the cooked salmon and drizzle over the sauce.

Aromatic Chicken Breast with Kale and Red Onions,Tomato and Chili Salsa

Ingredients:

120g skinless, boneless chicken breast

2 tsps. ground turmeric

juice of ¼ lemon

1 tbsp. extra virgin olive oil

50g kale, chopped

20g red onion, sliced

1 tsp. chopped fresh ginger

50g buckwheat

For the salsa

130g tomato (about 1)

1 bird's eye chili, finely chopped

1 tbsp. capers, finely chopped

5g parsley, finely chopped

Juice of ¼ lemon

Directions:

To produce the salsa, cut the tomato's eye and finely slice it, make sure to retain as much liquid as possible. Pair chili, capers, parsley, and lemon juice. You might place anything in a blender, but the end product is different.

Temperature up to 220°C / gas 7.

Marinate chicken breast in 1 turmeric tablespoon, lemon juice, and a little butter.

Heat the frying pan until soft, then attach the marinated chicken and cook for about a minute on each side until light yellow, then move to the oven (place on a baking tray if your pan is not ovenproof) for 8–10 minutes or until cooked through.

Remove from the oven, cover with foil for 5 minutes before eating.

In a steamer, cook the kale for 5 minutes.

Fry the red onions and ginger in a little oil until soft but not flavored, then add the cooked kale and fry for another minute.

Cook the buckwheat with the remaining turmeric tablespoon.

Serve rice, tomatoes, and salsa.

Greek Salad Skewers

Ingredients:

2 wooden skewers, soak for 30 minutes before use

8 cherry tomatoes

8 large black olives

1 yellow pepper, cut into 8 squares

100 g cucumber (approx. 10 cm), sliced into 4 pieces and halved

100g feta, cut into 8 cubes

½ red onion, cut in half and separated into 8 pieces

For the dressing:

1 tbsp. extra virgin olive oil

Juice of ½ lemon

1 tsp. balsamic vinegar

½ clove garlic, peeled and crushed

Few leaves basil, finely chopped (or ½ tsp. dried mixed herbs to replace basil and oregano)

Few leaves oregano, finely chopped

A good salt seasoning, and fresh black pepper

Directions:

Thread per skewer in the order: olive, tomato, yellow pepper, red onion, cucumber, feta, tomato, and olive, yellow pepper, red onion, cucumber, and feta.

Place all the ingredients and mix thoroughly in a bowl. Sprinkle over the sprouts.

5.4 Meals for Family

Breakfast

Sirtfood Mushroom Scramble Eggs

Ingredients:

2 eggs

1 tsp. ground turmeric

1 tsp. mild curry powder

20g kale, roughly chopped

1 tsp. extra virgin olive oil

½ bird's eye chili, thinly sliced

5g parsley, finely chopped

a handful of button mushrooms, thinly sliced

optional Add a seed mixture to taste and some rooster sauce

Directions:

Combine the turmeric and curry powder and apply water until you have a soft paste.

Steam kale 2–3 minutes.

Heat the oil over medium heat in a frying pan and cook the chili and mushrooms for 2–3 minutes until brown and soften.

Apple Pancakes with Blackcurrant Compote

Ingredients:

75g porridge oats

2 tbsp. caster sugar

125g plain flour

1 tsp. baking powder

2 Apples, peeled, chopped into small pieces

Pinch of salt

2 tsp. light olive oil

300ml semi-skimmed milk

2 egg whites

For the compote:

120g blackcurrants washed and stalks removed

2 tbsps. caster sugar

3 tbsp. water

Directions:

Render the compote first. Layer blackcurrants, sugar, and water in a cup. Simmer and simmer for 10-15 minutes.

Put in a big bowl, the peas, flour, baking powder, caster sugar, and salt. Cut the apple and stir in the milk until you have a nice mixture. Whisk the egg whites to firm peaks, then insert into the batter. Switch to a jar the hitter.

In a non-stick frying pan, heat 1/2 tsp. oil over medium-high heat and add roughly one-quarter of the batter—Cook golden brown on all ends. Undo to produce four pancakes.

Serve the blackcurrant compote-drizzled pancakes.

Sirty Blueberry Pancakes

Ingredients:

6 bananas

6 eggs

150g rolled oats

2 tsp. baking powder

¼ teaspoon salt

225g blueberries

Directions:

Pop the oatmeal in a high-speed blender and pump for 1 minute or until the oatmeal has developed. Tip: make sure your mixer is very dry before doing this, or else it's going to get soggy!

Add bananas, eggs, baking powder and salt to the blender and pulse until a smooth batter forms.

Switch the blueberries to a full bowl and fold. Leave the baking powder to rest for 10 minutes.

Apply a dollop of butter (this will render them moist and crispy!) to your frying pan at medium heat.

Add a few blueberry pancake spoons and fry to the bottom until nicely golden. Toss the pancake on the other side.

Enjoy it!

Vegetable Omelet

Ingredients:

2-3 organic eggs

2 Tbsp. olive oil

½ small onion, chopped

½ red pepper, chopped

Handful of fresh spinach

Sea salt

Directions:

Heat the olive oil over medium-high heat.

Begin cooking onions and peppers, then incorporate a few minutes later. When spinach wilts, put all vegetables in a small bowl.

In another cup, beat the eggs until combined. Add salt and pepper to taste. Add the eggs and spread them quickly around the pan.

After about a minute, add vegetables to half the omelet. Fold the omelet to cover vegetables. Slide the skillet onto your plate.

Season with salt again, and serve.

Lunch

Chinese-Style Pork with Pak Choi

Ingredients

400g firm tofu, cut into large cubes

1 tbsp. corn flour

1 tbsp. water

125ml chicken stock

1 tbsp. rice wine

1 tbsp. tomato purée

1 tsp. brown sugar

1 thumb (5cm) fresh ginger, peeled and sliced

1 tbsp. rapeseed oil

1 tbsp. soy sauce

1 clove garlic, peeled and crushed

1 shallot, peeled and sliced

100g shiitake mushrooms, sliced

200 g pak choi or Choi sum

400 g thin pork slices (10% fat)

100g beansprouts

Large handful (20g) parsley, chopped.

Directions:

Place tofu on kitchen paper, cover more kitchen paper, then put back.

Combine corn flour and water in a shallow tub, remove any lumps.

Add chicken, pasta, tomato purée, brown sugar, and soy sauce. Remove smashed garlic and ginger and mix.

Heat oil to high temperatures in a wok or large frying pan.

Add the shiitake mushrooms and stir-fry until cooked and shiny.

Pick mushrooms with a slotted spoon and put aside.

Add tofu and stir-fry until golden on both sides.

Set aside with a slotted spoon.

Add shallot and pak choi to the wok, stir-fry for 2 minutes, then apply to slim.

Cook until the thin is ready, then add the sauce, reduce the heat a notch and allow the sauce to bubble around the meat for a minute or two.

Add beansprouts, shiitake mushrooms, and tofu to the skillet and cook up.

Remove from oil, whisk through and serve immediately.

Fragrant Asian Hotpot

Ingredients:

1 tsp. tomato purée

1-star anise, crushed (or 1/4 tsp ground anise)

Juice of 1/2 lime

Small handful (10g) parsley, stalks finely chopped

50g broccoli, cut into small florets

50g cooked rice noodles according to packet instructions

1OOg raw tiger prawns

500ml chicken stock, fresh or made with 1 cube

Small handful (1Og) coriander, stalks finely chopped

1/2 carrot, peeled and cut into matchsticks

50g beansprouts

100g firm tofu, chopped

50g cooked water chestnuts, drained

20g sushi ginger, chopped

1 tbsp. good-quality miso paste

Directions:

Put the tomato purée, star anise, parsley stalks, coriander stalks, lime juice, and chicken stock in a big pan and simmer for 10 minutes.

Add cabbage, broccoli, prawns, tofu, noodles, and chestnuts and simmer gently before the prawns are finished. Remove from fire, apply sushi ginger and miso paste.

Serve with parsley and coriander seeds.

Kale, Edamame and Tofu Curry

Ingredients:

1 tbsp. rapeseed oil

1 large onion, chopped

4 cloves garlic, peeled and grated

1 large thumb (7cm) fresh ginger, peeled and grated

1 red chili, deseeded and thinly sliced

1/2 tsp. ground turmeric

1/4 tsp. cayenne pepper

1 tsp. paprika

1/2 tsp. ground cumin

1 tsp. salt

250g dried red lentils

1 liter boiling water

50g frozen soyaedamame beans

200g firm tofu, chopped into cubes

2 tomatoes, roughly chopped

Juice of 1 lime

200g kale leaves stalk removed and torn

Directions:

Place oil over low-medium heat in a heavy-bottom oven.

Add the onion and cook for 5 minutes before adding garlic, ginger, and chili, then cook for another 2 minutes. Add turmeric, cayenne, cinnamon, cumin, and oil.

Remove before inserting red lentils and mix them again.

Dump in boiling water, cook for 10 minutes, then rising heat and cook for another 20-30 minutes before the curry has a deep 'porridge' consistency.

Incorporate soybeans, tofu, tomatoes, and simmer for another 5 minutes.

Add lime juice and kale leaves and cook until soft.

Lamb, Butternut Squash and Date Tagine-

Ingredients:

2 tablespoons olive oil

1 red onion, sliced

2cm ginger, grated

3 garlic cloves, grated or crushed

1 teaspoon chili flakes (or to taste)

2 teaspoons cumin seeds

1 cinnamon stick

2 teaspoons ground turmeric

800g lamb neck fillet, cut into 2cm chunks

½ teaspoon salt

100g Medjool dates, pitted and chopped

400g tin chopped tomatoes, plus half a can of water

500g butternut squash, chopped into 1cm cubes

400g tin chickpeas, drained

2 tablespoons fresh coriander (plus extra for garnish)

Buckwheat, couscous, flatbreads or rice to serve

Directions:

Preheat oven to 140C.

Drizzle around 2 teaspoons of olive oil in a big, oven-proof casserole dish or cast iron. Add the sliced onion and cook over a gentle heat with the lid on until the onions are cooked but not dark.

Add garlic, ginger, chili, cumin, cinnamon, and turmeric. Take and cook the cover off for 1 minute. Apply water if it is too warm.

Add lamb pieces next. Apply oil, sliced dates, and tomatoes, plus about half a can of water (100-200ml) to cover the meat in the onions and spices.

Carry the tagine to the boil and place it on the cover for 1 hour and 15 minutes in your preheated oven.

Thirty minutes until the end of the cooking period, incorporate sliced butternut squash and chickpeas. Place the cover on and return to the oven for the remaining 30 minutes of cooking.

When the tagine is finished, extract the chopped coriander from the oven. Serve with buckwheat, couscous or basmati rice.

Notes:

If you don't possess an ovenproof casserole or cast iron casserole dish, just cook the tagine in a standard casserole before it needs to go into the oven and then move the tagine to a normal lidded casserole dish before putting in the oven. Add an additional 5 minutes cooking period to provide enough time to heat the casserole dish.

Dinner

Baked Potatoes with Spicy Chickpea Stew

Ingredients:

4-6 baking potatoes, pricked all over

2 tablespoons olive oil

2 red onions, finely chopped

4 cloves garlic, grated or crushed

2cm ginger, grated

½ -2 teaspoons chili flakes (depending on how hot you like things)

2 tablespoons turmeric

2 tablespoons cumin seeds

2 tablespoons unsweetened cocoa powder (or cacao)

Splash of water

2 yellow peppers (or whatever color you prefer!), chopped into bite size pieces

2 x 400 g tins of chickpeas (or kidney beans, if you prefer) plus don't drain.

2 x 400g tins chopped tomatoes

2 tablespoons parsley plus extra for garnish

Salt and pepper to taste (optional)

Side salad (optional)

Directions:

Preheat the oven to 200°C while preparing all your ingredients.

When the oven is hot enough, place the baked potatoes in the oven and cook for 1 hour or until they're finished like them.

Once the potatoes are in the oven, put the olive oil and diced red onion in a big broad saucepan and cook gently until the onions are soft but not dark.

Remove the cloth and add garlic, ginger, cumin, and chili. Cook on low heat for another minute, then add the turmeric and a very slight splash of water and cook for another minute, taking care not to dry the plate.

Add onions, chocolate powder (or coffee), chickpeas (including chickpea water), and yellow pepper. Take to boil, then cook 45 minutes on low heat until thick and unctuous (but don't let it burn!). The stew can be handled at the same time as potatoes.

Eventually, mix in 2 teaspoons of parsley and some salt and pepper, if needed, and serve the stew over the baked potatoes, or with a small side salad.

Turmeric Baked Salmon

Ingredients:

Skinned Salmon

1 tsp. Extra virgin olive oil

1 tsp. Ground turmeric

1/4 Juice of a lemon

1 tsp. Extra virgin olive oil

40 g Red onion, finely chopped

60 g Tinned green lentils

1 Garlic clove, finely chopped

1 Bird's eye chili, finely chopped

150 g Celery, cut into 2cm lengths

1 tsp. Mild curry powder

130 g Tomato, cut into 8 wedges

100 ml Chicken or vegetable stock

1 tbsp. Chopped parsley

Directions:

Heat the oven to 200°C / gas 6.

With the spicy celery. Prepare a saucepan over medium-low pressure, add olive oil, then onion, garlic, ginger, chili, and celery. For 2-3 minutes, fry gently, or until soft but not brown, apply the curry powder and fry for another minute.

Add the tomatoes and lentils and simmer gently for 10 minutes. You may want to raise or decrease cooking time, based on how crunchy the celery is.

Combine the turmeric, butter, and lemon juice and spray over the salmon. Put 8–10 minutes on a baking tray.

Stir the parsley through the celery and eat with salmon.

Bun-less Beef Burgers with All the Trimmings

Ingredients:

125 g Lean minced beef (5% fat)

15 g Red onion, finely chopped

1 tsp. Parsley, finely chopped

1 tsp. Extra virgin olive oil

150 g Sweet potatoes

1 tsp. Extra virgin olive oil

1 tsp. Dried rosemary

1 Garlic clove, unpeeled

10 g Cheddar cheese, sliced or grated

150 g Red onion, sliced into rings

30 g Tomato, sliced

10 g Rocket

1 Gherkin (optional)

Directions:

Temperature up to 220°C / gas 7.

Start by making fries. Split the sweet potato into 1 cm thick slices. Add olive oil, rosemary, and garlic clove. Put on a baking sheet and fry for 30 minutes until good, crispy.

Combine the onion and parsley with the ground beef. Whether you have pastry cutters, mold your burger with the set's largest pastry cutter, otherwise, just use your hands to produce a good even patty.

Steam a frying pan over medium heat, add olive oil, put the burger on one side of the pan, and rings on the other. Cook the burger on every side for 6 minutes, meaning it's finished. Fry the onion rings to your taste.

When the burger is baked, add the cheese and red onion and melt the cheese in the hot oven for a minute. Drop the onion, rocket, and gherkin. Serve the fries.

Chicken Skewers with Satay Sauce

Ingredients:

150 g Chicken breast, cut into chunks

1 tsp. Ground turmeric

1/2 tsp. Extra virgin olive oil

50 g Buckwheat

30 g Kale, stalks removed and sliced

30 g Celery, sliced

4 Walnut halves, chopped, to garnish

20 g Red onion, diced

1 Garlic clove, chopped

1 tsp. Extra virgin olive oil

1 tsp. Curry powder

1 tsp. Ground turmeric

50 ml Chicken stock

150 ml Coconut milk

1 tbsp. Walnut butter or peanut butter

1 tbsp. Coriander, chopped

Directions:

Combine the chicken with the turmeric and olive oil and put it aside to marinate - it'd be better for 30 minutes to 1 hour, so if you're low of time, keep it as long as you can.

Cook the buckwheat with the container instructions, incorporating the kale and celery for the last 5-7 minutes of the cooking time. Wash.

Steam the barbecue at high altitude.

Gently fry red onion and garlic in olive oil for 2-3 minutes until tender.

Add seasoning and cook another minute. Remove stock and coconut milk and curry to simmer, then incorporate butter and whisk. Reduce heat and simmer for 8-10 minutes, or until smooth and soft.

Thread the chicken on the skewers and put under the hot grill for 10 minutes, rotating after 5 minutes.

Stir the coriander through the sauce, pipe over the skewers, and sprinkle over the sliced walnuts.

Oriental Salmon & Broccoli Tray bake

Ingredients

Four skin-on salmon fillets

1 head broccoli broken into florets

juice ½ lemon

½ lemon quartered

small bunch spring onions sliced

2 tbsp. soy sauce

Directions:

Heat to 180°C/160°C fan or gas 4.

Place the salmon in a broad roasting pan, leaving filet with available space.

Wash and rinse broccoli and place the fillets in the tray while still a little dirty.

Pour lemon juice over both, then apply lemon pieces.

Drizzle with a little olive oil and place in the oven for 14 minutes.

Remove from the oven, sprinkle with soy, and return to the oven for 4 minutes until salmon is cooked through.

Sprinkle with remaining onions only before eating.

Chicken, Kale & Sprout Stir-Fry

Ingredients

100g soba noodle

100g shredded curly kale

2 tsp. sesame oil

2 lean skinless chicken breasts, sliced into thin strips

1 red pepper, deseeded and thinly sliced

25g piece fresh peeled ginger, sliced into matchsticks

1 tbsp. low-sodium soy sauce

handful Brussels sprout cut into quarters

2 tbsp. rice wine/white wine vinegar

Zest and juice 1 lime

Directions:

As instructed on the pack of noodles, cook the noodles, then drain and set aside.

In the meantime, heat a wide wok or frying pan, attach the kale with a decent splash of water, and cook for 1-2 minutes until it is wilted, then cool under running water to preserve the color.

Cook the chicken strips until browned, then cut and put aside.

Heat remaining oil and fry ginger, pepper, and sprouts until slightly softened. Save the chicken and the noodles.

Tip soy, rice wine, lime zest, and juice with ample water to make a sauce that clings to ingredients.

Immediately serve.

Chargrilled Beef with A Red Wine Jus, Garlic, Onion Rings, Kale and Herb Roasted Potatoes

Ingredients:

1 tbsp. extra virgin olive oil

100g peeled potatoes, cut into 2cm dice

50g red onion, sliced into rings

5g parsley, finely chopped

2cm-thick sirloin steak or 120–150g x 3.5cm-thick beef fillet steak

50g kale, sliced

1 tsp. tomato purée

1 garlic clove, finely chopped

150ml beef stock

40ml red wine

1 tsp. corn flour, dissolve it in 1 tbsp. water

Directions:

Temperature up to 220oC / gas 7.

Put the potatoes in a boiling water saucepan, carry back to boil and cook for 4–5 minutes, then drain.

Put 1 teaspoon of oil in a roasting pan and roast 35–45 minutes in the hot oven. Switch the potatoes to cook after 10 minutes. When baked, sprinkle with the minced parsley and blend well.

Fry the onion 5–7 minutes over medium heat in 1 tablespoon of butter, until smooth and caramel-like. Drain the kale for 2–3 minutes.

Fry the garlic in 1/2 teaspoon of oil for 1 minute, until tender, but not flavored. Add kale and fry for 1–2 minutes before tender. Keep dry.

Heat a frying pan over the high fire before burning. Coat the meat in 1/2 teaspoon of oil and fry over medium-high heat in the hot pan, depending on whether you prefer your meat.

When you want your meat mild, it will be easier to sear the meat and then move the pan to an oven set at 220oC / gas 7 and finish the cooking for the specified period.

Take the beef from the pan to cool. Attach the vinegar to the hot pan with any beef traces—bubble to halve the wine before syrupy with intense flavor.

Add the supply and tomato purée to the steak pan and bring to simmer, then attach the paste of corn flour to thicken the sauce, applying it a little at a time before you have a perfect consistency. Attach some of the resting steak juices and serve with grilled potatoes, spinach, onion rings, and red sauce.

5.5 Sirtfood Tea and Sweets Recipes

Sirtfood Tea Recipes:

Matcha with vanilla

INGREDIENTS:

½ tsp. matcha powder

Seeds from half a vanilla pod

DIRECTIONS:

Add 100 ml of water into a weighing container.

Place half the hot water in a shallow pot, then add the matcha powder and vanilla seeds to the container's remainder.

Whisk the mixture with a bamboo matcha whisk or mini electric whisk until smooth, lump-free, and bubbly. Discard the water in the teapot, then drink the cooked matcha tea.

Turmeric tea

INGREDIENTS:

3 heaped tsp. ground turmeric

1 tbsp. fresh grated ginger

1 small orange, zest pared

Honey/agave and slices of lemon slices to serve

DIRECTIONS:

Boil 500ml in the pot.

Place the turmeric, ginger, and orange in a teapot or bottle.

Pour over the boiling water for about 5 minutes.

Strain into two cups of sieve or tea strainer, and apply a slice of lemon and sweeten with honey or agave if you prefer.

Sweets:

Sirtfood Bites (Makes 15-20 Bites)

Ingredients:

120g walnuts

30 g dark chocolate (85% strong cocoa), cut into pieces; or cocoa nibs

Scraped 1 vanilla pod or 1 tsp. vanilla extract

1 tbsp. cocoa powder

250g Medjool dates pitted

1 tbsp. extra virgin olive oil

1-2 tbsp. water

1 tbsp. ground turmeric

Directions:

Put walnuts and chocolate in a food processor and heat until fine.

Remove all other ingredients except water, combine until the mixture forms a disc.

Depending on the mixture's thickness, you can or do not have to apply water - you don't want it to be so wet.

Shape the mixture into bite-sized balls and refrigerate in an airtight jar for at least 1 hour before feeding.

You should roll in any more cocoa or desiccated coconut to create a special finish if you prefer. They'll live up to 1 week in your fridge.

Chocolate Cupcakes with Matcha Icing

Ingredients:

150g self-rising flour

200g caster sugar

60g cocoa

½ tsp. salt

½ tsp. fine espresso coffee, decaf if preferred

120ml milk

½ tsp. vanilla extract

50ml vegetable oil

1 egg

120ml boiling water

For the icing:

50g butter, at room temperature

50g icing sugar

1 tbsp. matcha green tea powder

½ tsp. vanilla bean paste

50g soft cream cheese

Directions:

Preheat to 180C/160C fan. Line a paper or silicone cake cupcake tray.

Put flour, sugar, chocolate, salt, and espresso powder in a big pot, blend well.

Apply the butter, vanilla extract, vegetable oil, and egg to the dry ingredients and use an electric mixer to beat well.

Pour the boiling water steadily and beat at low speed before thoroughly mixed. Using a fast pace to smash the batter for another minute. It's much more liquid than a regular cake mix. Have confidence, awesome taste!

Batter spoon equally between cake cases. Cake case should be 3⁄4 complete. Bake 15-18 minutes in the oven before the mixture bounces when pressed. Remove and allow to cool fully until icing.

Cream butter and icing sugar together until soft and creamy. Stir the matcha powder and coffee. Apply cream cheese and beat until smooth. Pipe or scatter the sweets.

No-Bake Chocolate Coconut Energy Balls

Ingredients:

3/4 cup almonds, sliced or slivered

1/2 cup unsweetened cocoa

2 tablespoons ground flaxseed (use whole flax seeds and grind them yourself using a coffee grinder)

1/4 teaspoon ground sea salt

1 1/3 cups organic old fashioned rolled oats,

gluten-free if desired

1 pound (16-ounces) Medjool dates, pits

removed (if dates are not soft, soak them in water for 20 minutes first)

1/4 cup unrefined coconut oil, melted

1/4 cup finely shredded unsweetened coconut

Directions:

Add the almond slices to a food processor and cycle for 20-30 seconds before doing.

Add chocolate, flax, sea salt, and oats. Process another 20 seconds or so before combined.

Add dates, coconut oil. Process 2-3 minutes or before well blended. Note: you may need to stop, stir, and blend every 30 seconds again, depending on how sharp your blade is, so everything mixes equally.

The mixture would be solid enough to shape spheres. Test this by squeezing between your fingers. It should stay together, but not stick to or fall apart. If it doesn't stay together very well, add a little more coconut oil and re-process. If it's too sticky, add some oatmeal or even unsweetened coconut and re-blend. If set, shape 1 1/2 "balls. Note: If you think you can't really "roll" these between your hands to form the balls; you need to shape them, pressing with your hands until they're ball-shaped.

Place each ball on a plate or a baking sheet covered with parchment paper (or use a silicone baking mat). Any flat surface does.

Place finely sliced coconut on a different tray, cutting board, or another flat surface. Note: finely shredded fits well as well. Push each ball with a little energy, one by one, onto the coconut until it sticks on all sides. Airtight container transfer. Store in the fridge for a week. This recipe yields 22 cubes.

Chocolate coffee mousse

Ingredients:

Almond milk 300 ml

Coffee 200 ml

Gelatin powder 1 Tbsp

Maple syrup 2 Tbsp

Cinnamon 1/2 tsp

Chocolate pure (> 70% cocoa) 200 g

Coconut yogurt 300 g

Cocoa powder 2 Tbsp

Directions:

Combine almond milk and coffee in a casserole, sprinkle the gelatin over it, let stand for 5 minutes.

Bring the water to the boil quickly. Remove pan from heat immediately.

Stir in hot liquid maple syrup, cinnamon, and dark chocolate. Stir until the chocolate has fully melted and absorbed into the mixture.

Divide over decorative dessert glasses and place them in the fridge for at least 4 hours.

Garnish with almond milk and cocoa dust before eating.

Conclusion

Trendy new diets tend to crop up frequently, and one of the latest is the Sirtfood Diet.

It has become a favorite of Europe's celebrities and is known for allowing red wine and chocolate. Adele's incredible weight loss is thought to be behind the Sirtfood Diet.

Its creators insist that it's not a fad, but that "sirt foods" are the secret to unlocking fat loss and disease prevention.

Health experts, however, warn that this diet may not live up to the hype, and may even be a bad idea.

Sirtfood Diet was created by two celebrity nutritionists working with a private gym in the UK.

The Sirtfood Diet is focused on research into sirtuins, a group of proteins that control different body functions. Some foods called sirt foods might cause more of those proteins to be produced by the body. They promote the diet plan as a groundbreaking new health and diet plan that functions by turning your "skinny gene" on.

This diet is based on sirtuin research (SIRTs), a group of seven proteins found in the body that has been shown to regulate a variety of functions, including metabolism, inflammation, and lifespan;

The Sirtfood Diet is composed of two steps. Phase one lasts seven days, combining calorie restriction with green juices. Phase two lasts two weeks and consists of three meals and juice.

This diet will help with weight loss since its low in fat and calories, so after the diet begins, the weight would definitely return. The diet is too short to impact on your health over the long term.

The Sirtfood Diet is packed with healthier options, but eating patterns are not correct.

Its theory and health claims are, not to mention, based on enormous extrapolations from preliminary scientific evidence.

Although it isn't a terrible thing to attach any sirt products to the diet and might even provide specific health benefits, the diet itself seems like another fad.

Overall we can see the Sirtfood diet's advantages and appeal. As about every diet schedule, having all the ingredients can be a difficult task, and the 'Sirtfood Green Juice,' which forms a crucial part of the program's first 14 days, is unpleasant and very costly, but it tastes much better than you might imagine. While several other people have found a substantial weight drop in the trials, the book's pure gain is the smart way of incorporating Sirtfoods into your everyday meal schedule.

Consuming more sirtuin-rich foods is beneficial for your wellbeing, and you can quickly incorporate them into your diet without restricting yourself to one meal or one juice at a time. Eating more fish, berries, and leafy greens (mainly because these foods are packed with fiber and protein) and having a low-sugar green juice could be a great addition to an already balanced diet.

Ultimately, you'll be able to enjoy the advantages of the SIRT diet without fully jumping in. Just make sure your portions are sensible, and you get your calories from a wide range of healthy sources – no need for a crash diet or juice fasting.

Although not usually allowed at the pace people might typically prefer, the Sirt diet recipes are super yummy, filled with flavor, and satiating.

The meal plans are, at face value, relatively simple to adhere to - whether you have little better to do, be it exercising, socializing, dating, spending late nights, or meeting job obligations. The days you had to deal with all of those as mentioned above, the diet dropped apart. Like all other diets you've attempted (and struggled to) in the past, Sirt is fantastic in principle - on paper - but in reality, it might seem a little unrealistic for an authentic living, breathing, hungry human being.

There are several items that you can carry home - chopping milky lattes daily, incorporating more frequent green veggie drinks and avoiding snacks that travel at blinding speed through the tasty workplace meals. Yet when it comes to eating once or twice a day and feeding by 7 pm for those with a life beyond Sirt, the difficulty is not to adhere to the diet guidelines, but instead to find the opportunity to be on a diet within real life.

The allowed Sirtfood diet foods are low in calories and high in nutrients, which is ideal for losing weight. Although nutritionally speaking, this specific diet is stringent, which may make it impossible for particular individuals to follow. Talk to a doctor you trust, before you start, whether the plan is right for you.

Go ahead and consume more "sirtfoods," but then consider twice before you entirely stick to the Sirtfood Diet. Most dieticians and nutritionists believe that "sirt products" filled with plants and antioxidants will make a tremendously beneficial addition to your diet and help promote weight loss or proper weight maintenance. But as for the diet itself, there is no good science to suggest that it will activate your "skinny genes" or significantly affect sirtuins.

Any weight reduction from adopting a Sirtfood diet will possibly be chalked up to eating fewer calories, more nutrition, and ultimately absorbing more nutrients – which you could notice in any variety of dietary approaches. If you intend to pursue it, please ensure to have lots of good protein and fat (a Mediterranean-style diet bolstered with additional "sirtfoods" would be an excellent place to start), and consider consulting with a registered dietitian for help customizing a plan that's tailored for your specific needs and goals.

Sirtfood diet has left us all in a state of uncertainty and amazement due to its nuanced existence, but if we hold all aspects aside, there remains the safe side of sirtfood. In our everyday lives, we can easily integrate sirtfoods to maintain a balanced lifestyle.

Before beginning any diet program, the most important consideration is its effectiveness and suitability to our bodies, which is explored in-depth in this book and will help you make the right decision.

Lightning Source UK Ltd.
Milton Keynes UK
UKHW022046201220
375593UK00004B/89

9 781801 447034